100 Diagnostic Challenges
in Clinical Medicine

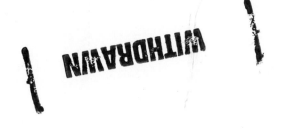

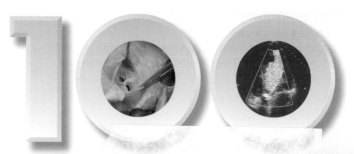

Diagnostic
Challenges

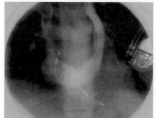

in Clinical
Medicine

David R Ramsdale
The Cardiothoracic Centre, UK

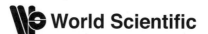

World Scientific

NEW JERSEY · LONDON · SINGAPORE · BEIJING · SHANGHAI · HONG KONG · TAIPEI · CHENNAI

Published by

World Scientific Publishing Co. Pte. Ltd.

5 Toh Tuck Link, Singapore 596224

USA office: 27 Warren Street, Suite 401-402, Hackensack, NJ 07601

UK office: 57 Shelton Street, Covent Garden, London WC2H 9HE

British Library Cataloguing-in-Publication Data
A catalogue record for this book is available from the British Library.

ISBN-13 978-981-283-939-8
ISBN-10 981-283-939-9
ISBN-13 978-981-4271-74-5 (pbk)
ISBN-10 981-4271-74-8 (pbk)

Typeset by Stallion Press
Email: enquiries@stallionpress.com

Printed by FuIsland Offset Printing (S) Pte Ltd, Singapore

*This book is dedicated to the many medical students
and junior doctors whom I have had the privilege to teach
over the last 30 years in preparation for their finals or higher
examinations. I hope those who are to follow in their footsteps
might enjoy reading this book and be stimulated by trying
to work out the clinical puzzles that are presented.*

Acknowledgements

I acknowledge the help from several colleagues who have kindly provided some of the case illustrations. These include Dr Derek Todd, Consultant Cardiologist and Electrophysiologist; Dr Norman Coulshed and Dr Ellis Epstein, Consultant Cardiologists; Dr Simon Modi, Specialist Registrar in Cardiology; Dr Charles Hind, Consultant Chest Physician; Dr Patrick Chu, Consultant Haematologist; Dr Martin Walshaw, Consultant Chest Physician; Dr Peter Humphrey, Consultant Neurologist and Janet Beukers, Senior Physiological Measurement Technician and Specialist in Echocardiography. I am also grateful to Drs Shahid Aziz and Archana Rao for their help in putting together some of the interesting cases in this book.

Preface

Good revision in preparation for important clinical examinations such as finals in medical school, entrance exams into the USA or membership exams for the Royal College of Physicians is essential if success is to be achieved. Although there can be no substitute for live revision courses involving real patients with a variety of clinical problems with good physical signs, further practice in diagnosis, planning investigations and treatment strategies can be obtained by trying to solve the well-illustrated case problems with accompanying clinical scenarios presented in this book. In this way, I hope that this book will prove to be useful revision for medical students preparing for finals and junior doctors who are preparing for their higher examinations and that it will provide enjoyment and a thirst for more knowledge!

David R. Ramsdale

Case 1

Following a syncopal episode at home, this 39-year-old man suffered from a fractured clavicle. He admitted to being breathless on effort and complained of difficulty in walking and poor vision. His facial appearance and his electrocardiogram (ECG) are shown below.

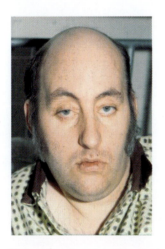

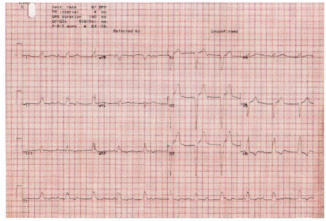

Questions:

1. What three features are shown in the picture?
2. What might explain his poor vision?
3. What is the clinical diagnosis? How is this condition inherited?
4. Which chromosome is abnormally affected?
5. What is the ECG diagnosis?
6. What precise treatment should he receive?

Answers:

1. Frontal balding, bilateral ptosis and long, haggard expressionless features.
2. Cataracts and external opthalmoplegia.
3. Dystrophia myotonica. Autosomal dominant.
4. Chromosome 19.
5. Complete heart block.
6. Dual chamber permanent pacemaker implantation.

Case 2

A 50-year-old lady complained of painful lower legs over the previous seven days. She had a four-year history of mild hypertension and a ten-year history of ulcerative colitis for which she received sulphasalazine.

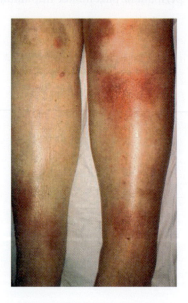

Questions:

1. Describe the lesions.
2. What is this condition? What is the pathology?
3. With what is it associated?
4. What is the usual outcome and what treatment could be given?

Answers:

1. Multiple raised red areas on the shins, which are tender.
2. Erythema nodosum. Panniculitis.
3. It may be associated with sarcoidosis, tuberculosis, rheumatic heart disease and streptococcal infection. It can also be seen in approximately 5% of patients with an exacerbation of inflammatory bowel disease. Females are affected three times more frequently than males. Drug hypersensitivity (e.g. oral contraceptives, penicillin) may be a cause as well.
4. Some severe lesions may ulcerate but are rarely chronic. They usually resolve with steroid therapy or after colectomy.

Case **3**

This 75-year-old man presented with cough and a large amount of haemoptysis. He had previously been treated for pulmonary tuberculosis with triple therapy and chronically expectorated large volumes of pale-green coloured sputum. In the last six months, the sputum had become progressively more blood stained.

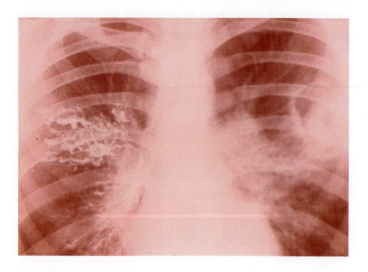

Questions:

1. Name three abnormalities on this chest X-ray.
2. What investigation has been performed here?
3. What is the diagnosis?
4. What simple tests might help confirm the diagnosis?
5. What treatment should be recommended?

Answers:

1. (i) Proximal bronchiectasis in right mid-zone.
    (ii) Bilateral hilar shadowing.
    (iii) Large cavitated lesion in left upper zone.
2. Bronchography.
3. Aspergilloma. The mycetoma is seen inside a large cavity in the left upper zone.
4. Fungal culture of sputum or bronchopulmonary lavage; serum IgG precipitins to *Aspergillus fumigatus*.
5. Left upper lobectomy with resection of mycetoma.

Case 4

A 60-year-man presented with angina of effort and exertional syncope. Physical examination revealed a small volume, anacrotic carotid pulse and an ejection systolic murmur at the left sternal edge. The left lateral chest X-ray and the M-mode echocardiogram are shown below.

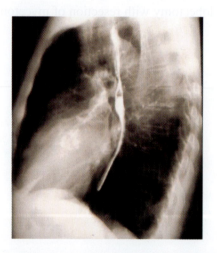

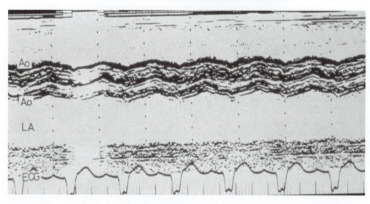

Questions:

1. What does the lateral chest X-ray show?
2. What does the M-mode echocardiogram show?
3. What is the diagnosis?
4. What is the next investigation required?
5. What treatment is indicated?

nswers:

1. A ring of calcification on the aortic valve.
2. Heavy (black) calcification on the aortic valve. (Ao = aorta; LA = left atrium)
3. Calcific aortic stenosis.
4. Cardiac catheterisation and coronary arteriography for assessment of the aortic valve gradient and the coronary anatomy.
5. Aortic valve replacement.

A 72-year-old man with a history of previous coronary artery bypass surgery and percutaneous coronary intervention to the saphenous vein grafts to the obtuse marginal branch of the circumflex artery and left anterior descending artery, complained of fatigue and dyspnoea of effort. He weighed 115 kg at 5 ft 10 in. Blood pressure was 140/80 mmHg, heart sounds were normal. Haemoglobin 11.6 g/dL; white cell count 20 000/μL; platelets 130 000/μL; ESR 40 mm in the first hour. The peripheral blood film is shown below.

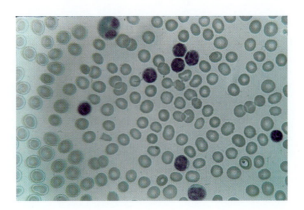

Questions:

1. What is the likely diagnosis?
2. Name the cell type.
3. What other clinical features should be looked for?
4. What two other investigations are indicated?
5. What treatment should be given?

Answers:

1. Chronic lymphatic leukaemia.
2. B cell.
3. Lymphadenopathy, splenomegaly.
4. Bone marrow aspiration, lymphocyte cell typing.
5. No specific treatment for the leukaemia at present, but needs regular follow-up by haematologist. Needs weight reducing diet.

This 55-year-old lady experienced weight loss and palpitations. She had suffered rheumatic fever during childhood and was diagnosed with pernicious anaemia five years earlier. She appeared anxious. The blood pressure was 150/85 mmHg, heart rate 110 bpm and irregular. Her fingers, legs and ECG are shown.

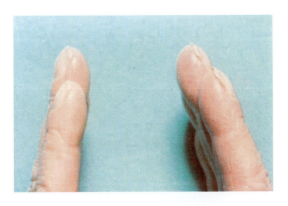
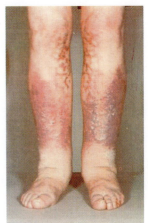

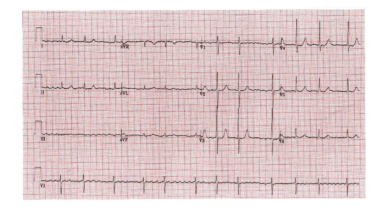

Questions:

1. What is the diagnosis?
2. What do the fingers show? What do the legs show?
3. What does the ECG show?
4. What four other clinical features might be evident?
5. What diagnostic tests should be requested?

Answers:

1. Hyperthyroidism — Graves' disease.
2. Thyroid acropachy — clubbing. Pretibial myxoedema — symmetrical, tender, itchy, purple-coloured, indurated lesions with well-defined serpiginous margins.
3. Atrial fibrillation.
4. Exophthalmos, lid retraction, lid lag, goiter, finger tremor.
5. (i) Thyroid function tests — high serum thyroxine and low TSH levels.
   (ii) Radioactive iodine uptake test — increased uptake.

A 26-year-old man was admitted with cough, chest pain and fever. He admitted to abusing cocaine and heroin for the past five years and there was evidence of two infected needle venepunctures on his left arm. On examination, he looked unwell. Temperature 38.3°C; pulse rate 115 bpm. Auscultation revealed a mid systolic murmur at the left sternal edge. The chest X-ray is shown.

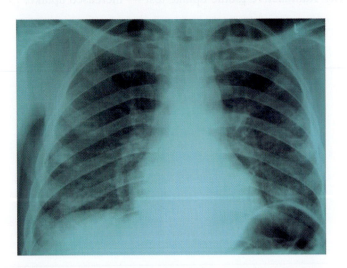

Q Questions:

1. What does the chest X-ray show?
2. What is the likely diagnosis?
3. What is the most common cause?
4. What three investigations should be performed?

Answers:

1. Lung abscesses are seen in both lungs. One in the right mid-zone and one in the left mid-zone appear to have fluid levels.
2. Tricuspid valve infective endocarditis due to IV drug abuse.
3. Staphylococcus septicaemia from infected needle injections is most probably responsible. Enterococci and fungi e.g. candida are less common causes.
4. (i) CAT scan.
   (ii) Blood cultures.
   (iii) Echocardiogram.

This 45-year-old woman complained of arthritis of her hands and Raynaud's phenomenon in her fingers. The second picture gives a clue to the diagnosis.

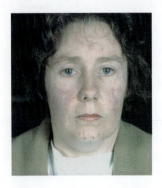 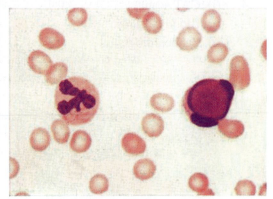

Questions:

1. What does the first picture show?
2. What is the diagnosis?
3. What does the second picture show?
4. How is the test performed?
5. What other clinical features would support the diagnosis?
6. What other tests might be consistent with the diagnosis?

Answers:

1. Malar "Butterfly" rash.
2. Systemic lupus erythematosus (SLE).
3. LE cell (right).
4. This film is made from the buffy coat of incubated defibrinated blood. The LE cell is a neutrophil containing a homogenous mass of basophilic material in its cytoplasm. When an injured neutrophil is exposed to the serum of a patient with SLE, the nucleus degenerates into a homogenous mass which is extruded and phagocyted by a healthy neutrophil.
5. Discoid skin rash, photosensitivity, mucous membrane ulcers, previous pleuritis/pericarditis, proteinuria or urinary casts, seizures or psychosis.
6. Antinuclear antibodies (95–98%). Anti–ds-DNA (anti-double strand DNA) (60–80%) or Anti-Sm antibodies (Sm is a ribonucleoprotein, found in nucleus) (30%), Anti-cardiolipin (anti-phospholipid) antibodies (33%).

Case 9

A 75-year-old retired cardiologist with a long history of systemic arterial hypertension suddenly developed expressive dysphasia one evening at the dinner table. The episode lasted five minutes and his speech returned to normal. Within 24 hours, he had two further episodes each lasting five minutes or so. Physical examination revealed BP 140/90 mmHg and a small fading bruise was visible on the side of his nose. There were no neurological signs. It was thought that he was having transient ischaemic attacks as a result of athero-sclerotic carotid disease and he was admitted with a view to heparinisation and antiplatelet therapy. A CT scan of the head was performed (shown below).

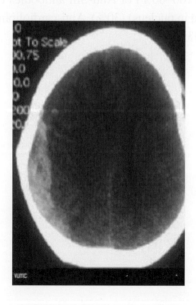

Questions:

1. What question should be asked?
2. What other diagnosis should be considered?
3. What does the CT scan show?
4. What treatment is indicated?

Answers:

1. Had he fallen and banged his head recently? In fact six weeks earlier, when visiting an old colleague at a local hotel, he had fallen down three stairs and banged his head on the wooden banister, breaking his spectacles. He did not lose consciousness.
2. Chronic subdural haematoma.
3. Subdural collection of blood in the left occipito-parietal area.
4. Burr-hole and surgical drainage.

A 17-year-old youth had a routine Football Association medical examination. He was found to have a systolic murmur at the second and third left intercostal spaces. The chest X-ray, echocardiogram and cardiac catheterisation data are shown.

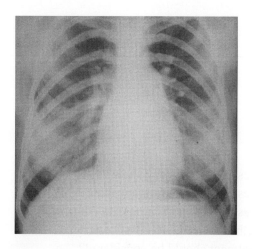

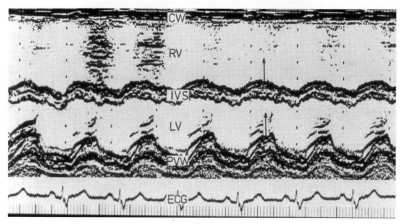

Cardiac catheterisation data:

Chamber	Pressures	Oxygen saturation
RA mid	mean 12 mmHg	85%
RV body	45/14 mmHg	86%
RV outflow		88%
PA	45/26 mean 34 mmHg	88%
LV	110/6 mmHg	99%
Ao	112/70 mmHg	99%
SVC		70%
IVC		65%
RA low		85%
RA high		88%

Questions:

1. What does the chest X-ray show?
2. What does the echocardiogram show?
3. What does the catheterisation data confirm?
4. What further investigation is necessary?
5. What treatment should be considered?

Answers:

1. Enlarged pulmonary conus and pulmonary plethora.
2. Dilated right ventricle (RV); paradoxical septal motion.
3. Step up in oxygen saturations from SVC/IVC into the right atrium confirms atrial septal defect. There is mild pulmonary artery hypertension.
4. 2-D transthoracic or transoesophageal echocardiography — to assess size and site of defect and its suitability for percutaneous closure.
5. Percutaneous or surgical closure.

Case 11

A 67-year-old man developed severe central chest pain when digging up a tree in his garden. The pain radiated up into his neck and down the left arm. He gave a history of hypertension, hypercholesterolaemia and previous smoking. BP was 170/110 mmHg; pulse 100 bpm; no cardiac murmurs were audible. The chest X-ray on admission, ECG (post-medical treatment) and CT scan (six hours later) are shown.

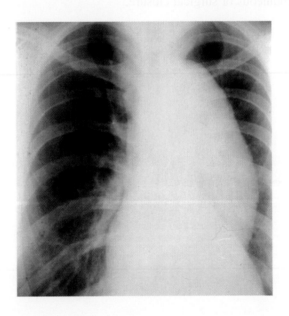

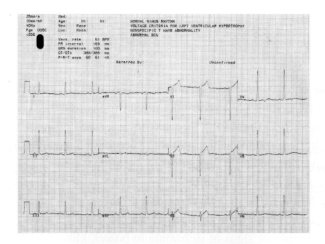

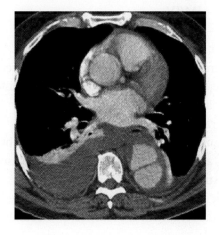

Questions:

1. What do the three illustrations show?
2. What is the diagnosis?
3. What other clinical features should be looked for?
4. What treatment should be given immediately?
5. What are the two most important investigations in such a patient?
6. What definitive treatment is indicated?

Answers:

1. The chest X-ray shows a widened mediastinum and thoracic aorta; the ECG shows left ventricular hypertrophy and the CT scan shows a dissection flap in the thoracic aorta as well as an effusion in the right hemithorax, which is almost certainly a haemothorax.
2. Type 1 acute aortic dissection.
3. Unequal or missing pulses.
   Different BP in the two arms.
   Signs of aortic regurgitation.
   Symptoms or signs of ischaemia to bowel, kidneys or lower limbs.
4. Analgesia — IM/IV.
   β-blocker — IV and oral to reduce BP.
   IV nitrate or nitroprusside to reduce BP.
5. (i) Echocardiography or CT scan. Both investigations showed that the tear originated in the ascending aorta, just above the aortic valve.
   (ii) Aortography — not done in this case.
6. Type 1 (intimal tear occurs in ascending aorta but extends into the descending aorta) and Type 2 (tear limited to ascending aorta) dissection — **surgical repair**.
   Type 3 (tear limited to descending aorta) — medical treatment initially; surgical treatment if evidence of bleeding e.g. haemothorax.

Case **12**

A 76-year-old vagrant was found semi-conscious in an alley on Christmas Eve with a bottle of methylated spirits by his side. His rectal temperature was 31°C and his body was covered in lice. He looked pale and cachectic. BP was 75/45 mmHg; pulse 35 bpm; heart sounds normal/quiet. Respiratory examination revealed poor air entry with crepitations in the right upper and mid zones. ECG showed sinus bradycardia. The chest X-ray is shown below.

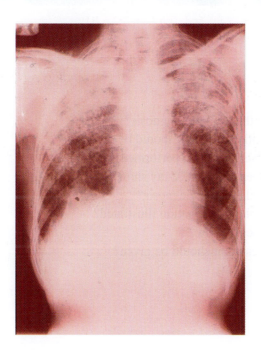

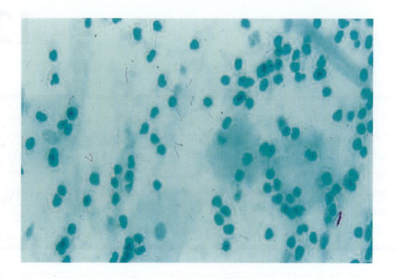

Questions:

1. What is the primary diagnosis?
2. What initial treatment should be offered?
3. What tests should be performed?
4. What does the chest X-ray show?
5. What is the likely diagnosis?
6. What is the investigation illustrated?
7. What does it show?
8. What treatment should be given?

Answers:

1. Hypothermia.
2. He should be washed, dusted with the insecticide DDT (Dichlorodiphenyltrichloroethane) powder, wrapped in a space blanket and given intravenous fluids. Rewarming should be gradual and the head covered. IV antibiotics e.g. amoxicillin should be commenced.
3. Blood count, electrolytes, blood glucose, liver function tests, thyroid function tests, ECG and chest X-ray. Blood and urine cultures (40% have sepsis or bacteraemia). Once stable, perform CT scan of head.
4. Bilateral upper zone shadows with cavitation in the left upper lobe and tenting of the right hemidiaphragm.
5. Pulmonary tuberculosis.
6. Ziehl–Neelsen stain on sputum sample.
7. Red stained rods of *Mycobacterium tuberculosis.*
8. Two months initial treatment with a combination of isoniazid/rifampicin/pyrazinamide and ethambutol, followed by six months of isoniazid and rifampicin.

A 51-year-old asthmatic man became unwell 24 hours after arriving in Barbados from the UK. He complained of a sore throat and neck, profound asthenia and had generalised aches and arthralgia with a temperature of 38°C. He was given antibiotics by a local doctor but there was little improvement despite a second course. After two weeks, he returned to the UK still feeling unwell. After a third antibiotic he felt slightly better and returned to work, when he suddenly developed rapid palpitations and dizziness. The ECG done at the local hospital is shown. After a failed cardioversion, intravenous amiodarone reverted him to sinus rhythm. Blood tests revealed: haemoglobin 14 g/dL; white cell count 8000/μL; platelets 450 000/μL. ESR 90 mm in first hour; CRP 25 mg/dL. Sodium 138 mmol/L; potassium 4.0 mmol/L; urea 6.4 mmol/L; creatinine 93 mmol/L. Free T4 55 pmol/L; TSH < 0.003 mU/L.

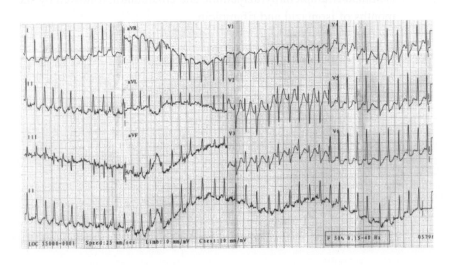

Questions:

1. What does the ECG show?
2. What is the likely diagnosis?
3. What other tests should be performed?
4. What treatment should be given?

Answers:

1. Rapid atrial fibrillation.
2. Acute thyroiditis — hyperthyroidism.
3.   (i) Radioactive thyroid uptake scan — should be depressed (elevated in Graves' disease).
     (ii) Thyroid autoantibodies — antithyroglobulin antibody and antithyroid peroxidase (anti-TPO or antimicrosomal) antibody.
     (iii) Blood cultures — in case of bacterial thyroiditis.
     (iv) Needle biopsy of thyroid.
4. Carbimazole 15 mg tds for 4–6 weeks; follow-up thyroid function tests with view to reducing dose. Flecainide 50 mg tds to maintain sinus rhythm and prevent return to atrial fibrillation.

   In severe cases, prednisolone (20–40 mg/day) may be necessary.

A 67-year-old man with obstructive airways disease had had coronary artery bypass (CABG) surgery to the left anterior descending (LAD), right (RCA) and obtuse marginal branch of the circumflex (OMCX) coronary arteries 15 years earlier. He presented with recurrent angina of effort limiting to 20 yards of effort. Despite aspirin, atenolol, isosorbide mononitrate and amlodipine, his symptoms deteriorated. Physical examination was unremarkable.The cardiologist performed coronary angiography which showed that the LAD and the RCA were occluded as was the saphenous vein graft to the OMCX. The LIMA to the LAD was fully patent. Two other coronary injections are shown below.

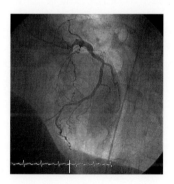 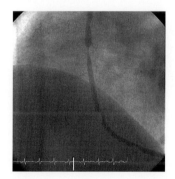

Questions:

1. What do the angiograms show?
2. What two treatments could be offered?
3. What treatment should be preferred?

Answers:

1. The left-hand angiogram shows a severe stenosis in the distal LCX coronary artery. The right-hand angiogram shows two moderately severe stenoses in the SVG to the RCA.
2. Percutaneous coronary intervention with stenting (PCI) to the distal LCX and SVG RCA lesions or repeat CABG surgery.
3. PCI should be preferred. The procedure is less invasive and carries less morbidity and mortality than repeat CABG surgery (< 1% vs. 2–6%).

These are the hands of a 62-year-old man.

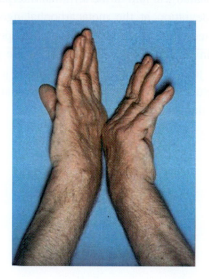

Questions:

1. What is this called?
2. What is it due to?
3. What is the anatomical explanation for the deformity?
4. Name two other hand deformities that may be seen in such patients.

Answers:

1. Swan-neck deformity of the proximal interphalangeal joints.
2. Rheumatoid arthritis.
3. Due to hyperextension of this joint with fixed flexion of the metacarpophalangeal and of the terminal interphalangeal joint.
4. (i) Ulnar deviation at the metacarpophalangeal joints — often associated with palmar subluxation of the proximal phalanges.
   (ii) Boutonnière (buttonhole) deformity of the proximal interphalangeal joint — flexion deformity of this joint with extension contracture of the metacarpophalangeal and of the terminal interphalangeal joint.

This 23-year-old man complained of feeling unwell with severe fatigue, muscle aches, sore throat and a painful neck and pain in the left side of his abdomen. On examination, he had a temperature of 38.3°C and bilateral cervical lymphadenopathy. The appearance on throat examination is shown. White cell count 15 000/μL. The peripheral blood film showed a preponderance of enlarged atypical lymphocytes, suggestive of lymphocytic or monocytic leukaemia. Liver function tests showed an ALT of 69 IU/L and bilirubin of 30 μmol/L.

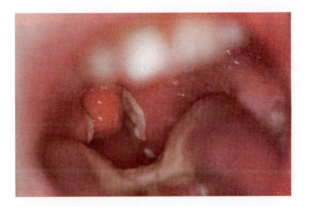

Questions:

1. What is the likely diagnosis?
2. What does the picture show?
3. What may be the cause of his abdominal pain?
4. What three tests are indicated?
5. Name three complications that may occur.

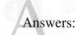Answers:

1. Infectious mononucleosis or glandular fever.
2. White exudates covering the tonsils.
3. Splenomegaly, which was indeed subsequently detected.
4. Throat swab for microscopy, culture and sensitivity testing. Heterophile IgM antibody titre of > 40-fold will be present in 40% in the first week and in 80–90% during the third week. This may be commercially available as a monospot test: Epstein-Barr Virus (EBV) specific antibodies e.g. anti-VCA IgM or IgG (antibodies to viral capsid antigen) — which will be present in > 90% at the onset of disease. In this case with severe uvula and pharyngeal swelling, *Streptococcus sanguis* was also identified from the throat swab and required penicillin treatment.
5. Upper airway obstruction due to inflammation/oedema of epiglottis, pharynx or uvula. Hepatitis, myocarditis, meningitis, encephalitis, splenic rupture, autoimmune haemolytic anaemia and long-lasting fatigue/tiredness/weakness and depression.

Case 17

This 78-year-old woman developed very itchy blisters on her limbs and abdomen. Two small blisters were noticed inside her mouth. The lesions on her abdomen and direct immunofluorescence histology are shown.

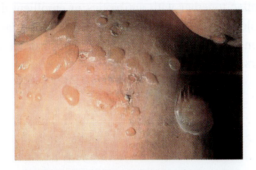

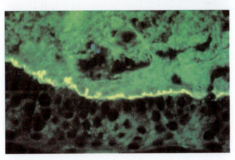

Questions:

1. What is the diagnosis?
2. What does the immunohistology show?
3. What treatment can be offered?

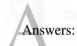

Answers:

1. Bullous pemphigoid.
2. IgG deposition in the epidermal basement membrane. Biopsies of inflammatory lesions typically show an eosinophil-rich, leukocytic infiltrate within the papillary dermis at sites of vesicle formation and in perivascular areas.
3. Local treatment includes aseptic puncture and collapse of the large tense bullae together with antibiotics or emollient dressings. Oral prednisolone (40–60 mg/day initially) in decreasing doses as remission occurs is usually prescribed. The disorder may persist for 1–5 years.

Case **18**

This young girl shows two typical features of an uncommon condition.

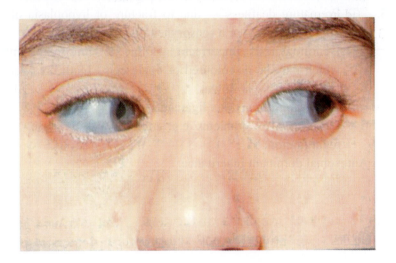

Questions:

1. What is the likely condition? How common is it?
2. What two features are apparent?
3. What other features are associated with the syndrome?
4. How is it inherited?

Answers:

1. Type 1 Osteogenesis Imperfecta. This is a true inherited collagen disorder. Its incidence is between 1 in 20 000 and 1 in 50 000 births.
2. Blue sclerae and arcus juvenilis. The former is attributed to thin sclerae which allows visibility of the pigmented choroid coat.
3. (i) Premature deafness — due to fracture or hypoplasia of the auditory ossicles or a sensoryneural defect.
    (ii) Dentinogenesis imperfecta — due to abnormal dentine which may be discoloured or opalescent. Teeth break easily and quickly wear down.
    (iii) Hypermobility and lax ligaments.
    (iv) Cardiac valve problems e.g. mitral valve prolapse, aortic regurgitation.
4. Autosomal dominant inheritance.

A 35-year-old female was admitted with a two-week history of progressively severe colicky abdominal pain, vomiting and constipation. She had had three previous admissions with similar symptoms and "chronic appendicitis" had been postulated as the likely diagnosis. For ten days she had noticed discomfort in the right arm, with clumsiness and weakness of the right arm and hand and some unsteadiness of gait.

On examination, she was mildly tender over her abdomen, particularly in the right iliac fossa but there was no guarding or rebound tenderness present. Temperature 37.5°C; heart rate 100 bpm; heart sounds were normal. Neurological examination suggested genuine loss of power in the right arm and diminished biceps and supinator tendon reflexes. Laboratory tests revealed haemoglobin 11.8 g/dL; white cell count 12 000/μL; bilirubin 8 mmol/L; sodium 140 mmol/L; potassium 3.9 mmol/L; urea 5.0 mmol/L; creatinine 98 mmol/L. Routine urine testing by the laboratory was reported as showing dark red urine but no red blood cells, leucocytes, haemoglobin or microorganisms were identified. Further laboratory testing on the urine is shown below.

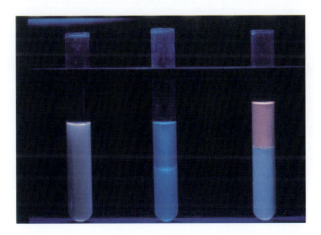

Q

Questions:

1. What test has been done on the urine?
2. What is present in the urine?
3. What is the likely diagnosis and what is the cause of the condition?
4. What other investigations should be performed?
5. What treatment can be offered?

Answers:

1. Urine has been mixed with an organic solvent and placed under ultra-violet (UV) light.
2. Porphyrins. The presence of porphyrins in the urine is shown by the red fluorescence in the upper layer under UV light.
3. Acute intermittent porphyria due to deficiency of the enzyme porphobilinogen deaminase.
4. Urine porphobilinogen and aminolaevulinic acid levels.
   CAT scan of head and abdomen.
5. There is no specific treatment that will abort an acute attack, but any drug that may be responsible for the acute attack should be stopped and the patient warned of the danger of subsequent use. Hemin (USA) and haem arginate (UK) may be effective in shortening an attack if administered early. These heme-like substances inhibit ALA synthase and hence the accumulation of toxic precursors. Alcohol excess and the contraceptive pill should be avoided.

A 52-year-old man was admitted with crushing central chest pain of six hours duration which began on the golf course. He was admitted to hospital as an emergency. He was sweating profusely. BP 110/70 mmHg; heart rate 130 bpm. His ECG is shown.

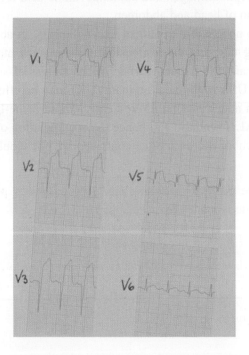

Twenty four hours later he became acutely breathless and hypotensive, BP 80/50 mmHg and developed a persistent tachycardia. Urine output fell to 30 ml/min and a pan systolic murmur was audible over the praecordium. The jugular venous pressure appeared to be elevated 4 cm above the sternal angle. The ECG showed atrial fibrillation and he was given IV digoxin. The chest X-ray is shown.

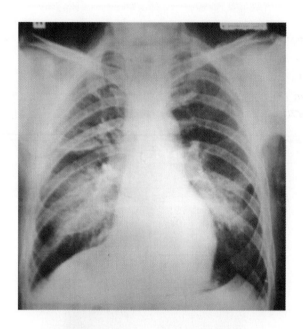

To confirm the diagnosis, cardiac catheterisation was performed. The following haemodynamic data was obtained:

SVC		sat: 75%			
RA	10 mmHg	sat: 75%	RV	44/14 mmHg	sat: 76%
PA	45/23 mmHg	sat: 77%	r PA	45/23 mmHg	sat: 76%
pcw (mean)	19 mmHg		LV	80/21 mmHg	sat: 93%
Ao	82/53 mmHg	sat: 94%			

Two simultaneous intracardiac pressures and the left ventricular angiogram are shown.

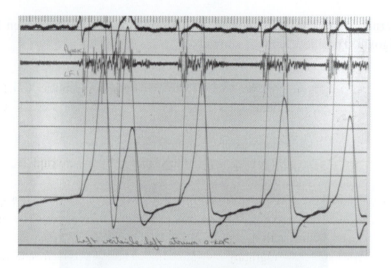

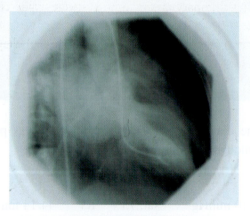

Q Questions:

1. What treatment was indicated on presentation?
2. What are the two differential diagnoses 24 hours later?
3. What immediate investigation should then be performed?
4. What is the diagnosis?
5. What other diagnostic information is necessary?
6. What treatment is required?

Answers:

1. Aspirin 600 mg orally stat; 5–10 mg diamorphine IV/IM; Thrombolytic therapy IV stat; IV heparin; admitted to CCU for observation.
2. (i) Acute ventricular septal rupture/defect.
   (ii) Acute mitral regurgitation due to papillary muscle rupture.
3. Echocardiography.
4. Acute mitral regurgitation due to papillary muscle rupture — shown by a large "V" wave in the left atrial trace; and the left atrium filling with contrast during left ventricular systole.
5. Coronary arteriography — showed an occluded left anterior descending coronary artery and a severe right coronary artery stenosis.
6. Intraaortic balloon counterpulsation and emergency mitral valve replacement plus coronary artery bypass surgery.

Case **21**

This 53-year-old lady was referred to clinic with a 12 month history of increasing breathlessness and substernal chest discomfort. The symptoms were exacerbated by exercise. She had recently lost 3 kg in weight without any obvious explanation. Past medical history revealed hypertension for five years, treated with nifedipine retard 30 mg od; pernicious anaemia diagnosed 11 years earlier and treated with monthly Vitamin B12 injections. She was receiving simvastatin 20 mg od for hypercholesterolaemia (total cholesterol 7.8 mmol/L; LDL 4.1 mmol/L) and she smoked 20 cigarettes per day.

Physical examination was unremarkable. The ECG was normal. The chest X-ray is shown.

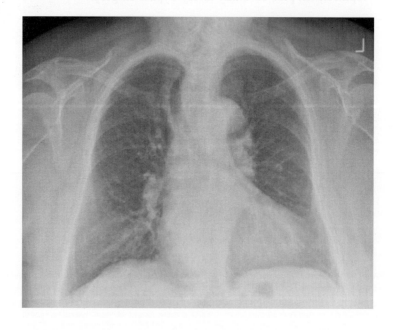

Questions:

1. What does the chest X-ray show?
2. What is the likely diagnosis?
3. What three further investigations are indicated?
4. What treatment should be offered?

Answers:

1. Marked deviation of the trachea to the right; superior mediastinal shadow.
2. Superior mediastinal mass — probably retrosternal thyroid.
3. (i) CAT scan of thorax.
    (ii) Thyroid function tests including radioisotope thyroid scan.
    (iii) Coronary angiography. This revealed left main stem stenosis as well as severe left anterior descending and left circumflex coronary artery stenoses.
4. Surgical removal of mass. This was done at the same time as coronary artery bypass surgery via a median sternotomy.

This 19-year-old student developed this rash on both hands and fore-arms with three similar lesions on the face and an ulcer on his lower lip. He was recovering from a mild upper respiratory tract infection and there was a crusted "cold sore" on the corner of his mouth.

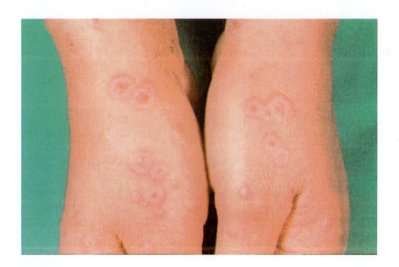

Questions:

1. What is this rash called?
2. Give three causes of this rash.
3. What treatment is necessary?

Answers:

1. Erythema multiforme.
2. (i) Viral infections.
    (ii) Drugs e.g. salicylates, gold.
    (iii) Post-radiotherapy.
3. Symptomatic/supportive e.g. local calamine lotion, antihistamines.

> *This peripheral blood film is from a febrile patient who has just returned from a holiday in Indonesia.*

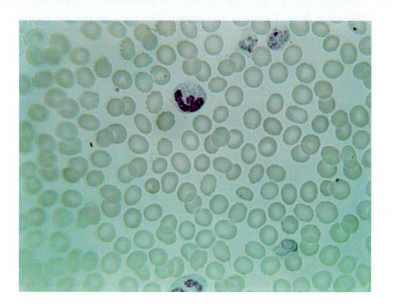

Questions:

1. What does the blood film show?
2. What is the diagnosis?
3. What is the main treatment for this condition?

Answers:

1. The blood film shows ring-form trophozoites within erythrocytes (top right quadrant).
2. Malaria due to infection with *Plasmodium vivax.*
3. Chloroquine or mefloquine. However, chloroquine resistance is common (up to 20% resistance) in Indonesia's Irian Jaya region (Western New Guinea) and artesunate may be the drug of choice (not approved in USA).

Case 24

An 18-year-old man was found to have hypertension (BP 185/105 mmHg) during a routine medical examination prior to Army recruitment. He was not on any medical treatment. His ECG and chest X-ray are shown.

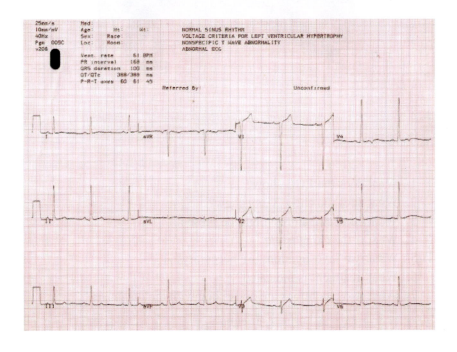

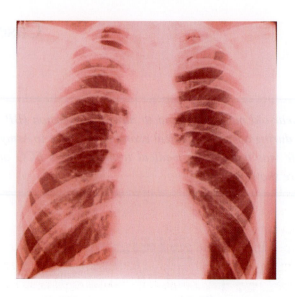

Questions:

1. What does the ECG show?
2. What does the chest X-ray show?
3. What clinical features might be present?
4. What is the diagnosis?
5. What two investigations are necessary?
6. What treatment is indicated?
7. What two conditions are associated with the diagnosis?

Answers:

1. Sinus rhythm. Voltage criteria for left ventricular hypertrophy.
2. Bilateral rib notching. Normal heart size.
3. Weak or impalpable femoral pulses.
   Radio-femoral delay.
   Palpable arterial pulsation over the scapulae.
   Systolic murmur over praecordium and over back.
4. Coarctation of the aorta.
5. Echocardiography; cardiac catheterization including aortography and an assessment of gradient across the coarctation.
6. Surgical resection with end-to-end anastomosis or tube graft inter-position depending on anatomy. Balloon dilatation and stenting may be an alternative.
7. Bicuspid aortic valve and cerebral "berry" aneurysms.

This 26-year-old Asian man developed left-sided facial pain and erythema four days after feeling generally unwell with a pyrexia of 37.8°C. Small, fluid-filled blisters appeared as the pain became intense and persistent but they ruptured and dried up. He developed severe pain in his left eye with a vesicle on the cornea. The picture shows his face eight days after the rash first appeared.

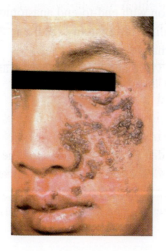

Questions:

1. What is the diagnosis?
2. What is the anatomical explanation for the distribution?
3. What neurological complication can occasionally accompany this condition?
4. What treatment can be offered?

Answers:

1. Opthalmic Herpes zoster (Shingles).
2. Acute infection of the posterior root ganglion by H. zoster with vesicles appearing in the cutaneous distribution of the root i.e. the opthalmic division of the fifth cranial nerve/trigeminal ganglion. When the tip of the nose is involved (Hutchinson's sign), there is a 75% chance of eye infection because of the involvement of the nasal branch of the nasociliary branch of the opthalmic division of the trigeminal nerve. In fact all skin lesions at the tip, the side and the root of the nose, representing the dermatomes of the external nasal and infratrochlear branches of the nasociliary nerve carry the same ocular potential in patients with herpes zoster opthalmicus.
3. Localised paralysis may accompany zoster. Third nerve palsy with ptosis and squint may occur. Chronic severe spontaneous facial pain or distressing hyperaesthesia can be so bad as to cause depression, anxiety and analgesia dependence.
4. If the diagnosis is made within 72 hours of onset, antiviral drugs such as acyclovir, famciclovir and valaciclovir might reduce the severity of the disease and even reduce the duration of post-herpetic neuralgia. Corticosteroids should be used as soon as the diagnosis is made. Vesicles should be kept dry and calamine lotion may provide some local relief. Analgesia is invariably necessary.

This patient complained of painful fingers and toes and severe low back pain. The distal aspects of the fingers are shown.

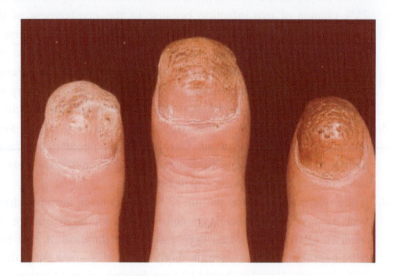

Questions:

1. What is the diagnosis?
2. Name three features that are shown.
3. What other clinical evidence might clinch the diagnosis?
4. What is the likely cause of the back pain?
5. What three tests are indicated?

Answers:

1. Psoriatic arthropathy.
2. (i) Thimble-like pitting of the nail plate. Thickening of nail plate (subungual hyperkeratosis).
   (ii) Yellow/browny-red discoloration of nail — termed "salmon patch". Onycholysis (lifting of nail).
   (iii) Swollen distal interphalangeal joints.
3. Presence of psoriasis of the skin.
4. Sacroiliitis or spondylitis.
5. (i) X-ray of hands and feet for erosive arthropathy of the distal interphalangeal joints and florid periosteal proliferation. "Pencil-in-cup" and "opera-glass" deformity are typical features.
   (ii) X-ray of sacroiliac joints for asymmetric or unilateral sacroiliitis.
   (iii) Serum rheumatoid factor — usually negative.

This 37-year-old man presented to his general practitioner with symptoms of headache, tiredness, impotence and depression. Over the past eight months he had put on 15 kg in weight and reported thirst and polyuria. On examination, he had a rounded face which appeared purple or plum-coloured. There was marked truncal obesity and striae were visible around his hips and flanks. His blood pressure was 180/110 mmHg and glycosuria was present on routine urine testing.

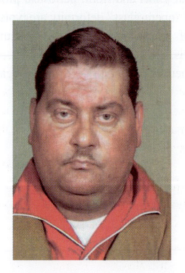

Questions:

1. What is the likely diagnosis? What is the pathology?
2. What three tests would confirm the diagnosis?
3. What treatment should be offered?

Answers:

1. Cushing's syndrome. Bilateral cortical adrenal hyperplasia due to hypersecretion of pituitary ACTH.
2.   (i) Elevated plasma cortisol at midnight.
    (ii) Elevated 24-hour urinary free-cortisol level (> 100 micrograms).
    (iii) Dexamethasone suppression tests. The best screening procedure is the overnight Dexamethasone suppression test. This involves the measurement of plasma cortisol levels at 8 am following the oral administration of 1 mg of Dexamethasone the previous midnight. The 8 am plasma cortisol in normal subjects should be < 140 nmol/L. The definitive test of adrenal suppressibility consists in administering 0.5 mg Dexamethasone every six hours for two successive days while collecting urine over a 24-hour period for determination of creatinine and free cortisol and/or measuring plasma cortisol levels. In a patient with a normal hypothalamic-pituitary ACTH release mechanism, a fall in the urine free cortisol to less than 80 nmol/L or plasma cortisol to less than 140 nmol/L will be seen on the second day.
    (iv) Serum level of ACTH.
        CRH (corticotropin-releasing hormone) stimulation test can help distinguish between those with pituitary adenomas and those with ectopic ACTH-production from tumours e.g. lung, medullary thyroid tumours.
    (v) CT and/or MRI imaging to search for source of tumour e.g. pituitary, adrenal or ectopic source.
3. Bilateral adrenalectomy with cortisone and fludrocortisone replacement therapy. If a pituitary ACTH-producing adenoma can be proven, then removal or hypophysectomy should be performed. For those unfit for surgery, medical adrenalectomy using ketoconazole, mitotane, aminoglutethimide or metyrapone may be used.

A 78-year-old woman collapsed whilst attending a birthday party, fracturing her left clavicle. She gave a history of hypertension and diabetes. Physical examination revealed an ejection systolic murmur over the second right intercostal space. Medication included ramipril 2.5 mg/day, aspirin 75 mg/day and gliclazide 80 mg bd. The ECG on arrival at hospital is shown uppermost.

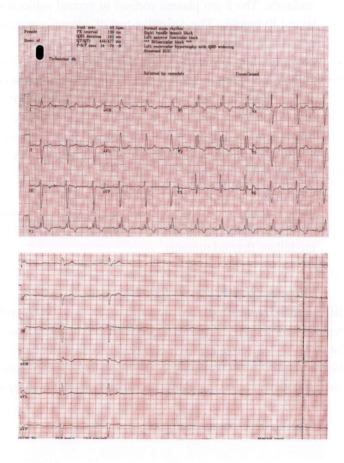

Questions:

1. What is the diagnosis?
2. What other two diagnoses should be considered?
3. What clinical test has been performed at the bedside?
4. What do the ECGs show?
5. What other tests should be arranged with some urgency?
6. What treatment is indicated?

Answers:

1. Carotid sinus hypersensitivity/sick sinus syndrome and conduction tissue fibrosis.
2. Aortic stenosis; hypotension due to ACE inhibitor.
3. Carotid sinus massage was performed at the bedside whilst an ECG was being recorded (lowermost ECG) and produced prolonged asystole and the beginnings of a Stokes–Adams attack.
4. The top ECG shows bifascicular block (right bundle branch block and left axis deviation). The bottom ECG shows prolonged sinus arrest and ventricular asystole.
5. Echocardiogram and CT scan of head.
6. Dual chamber (DDD) or A-V sequential pacemaker implantation.

Case 29

A 36-year-old woman presented with a 12 month history of progressive tiredness, fatigue and malaise. She had experienced episodes of feeling faint and sweaty. Her appetite had diminished and she had lost 1 stone in weight over the past six months. Her relatives commented that she looked well with a good skin tan and wondered whether stress in her personal life was the cause of her symptoms although she denied any family or emotional problems. She had had asthma in childhood. Pernicious anaemia was diagnosed four years earlier and this was treated by vitamin B12 injections. On examination, she looked tanned and slim. BP 110/65 mmHg; heart rate 80 bpm. There were no abnormalities on examining the respiratory and cardiovascular systems. All reflexes were present and equal although the ankle jerks seemed slightly sluggish. Her hands are shown.

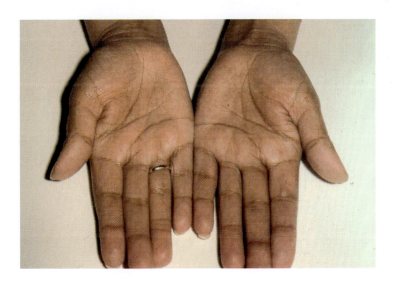

Q

Questions:

1. What do the hands show?
2. What is the diagnosis?
3. What three diagnostic tests are indicated?
4. What treatment is required?
5. What important instruction should be given to the patient?

Answers:

1. Pigmentation of the palmar creases.
2. Addison's disease or chronic adrenal insufficiency. Causes include: Autoimmune destruction of adrenal cortex, adrenoleukodystrophy, infections (TB, histoplasmosis), haemorrhage (Waterhouse–Friderichsen syndrome), metastatic disease.
3. (i) Plasma cortisol (usually insufficient on its own).
   (ii) ACTH stimulation test.
   (iii) 24 hr urinary 17-hydroxycorticosteroid excretion low.
   (iv) CT and/or MRI scan might help to determine the aetiology.
4. Oral hydrocortisone and fludrocortisone acetate.
5. She should be given a card or bracelet to always carry with her, which indicates the diagnosis and the need for increased glucocorticoid dosage in the event of intercurrent infection, trauma or psychological disturbance.

This 57-year-old man complained of bloody sputum. He had twice undergone coronary artery bypass surgery 18 years and 8 years earlier. He had also undergone multiple percutaneous coronary intervention procedures to saphenous vein graft disease and was currently having mild angina pectoris on medication. His medication included aspirin 75 mg/day, atenolol 50 mg/day, nifedipine retard 20 mg/day and simvastatin 20 mg/day. There were no abnormalities on physical examination except for this appearance in the mouth.

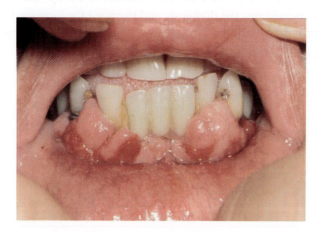

Questions:

1. What is this condition?
2. What is the likely cause?
3. What other causes are there?
4. What treatment is required?

Answers:

1. Gingival hyperplasia/hypertrophy.
2. Nifedipine.
3. Other calcium antagonists e.g. amlodipine, diltiazem, verapamil.
   Phenytoin, phenobarbitone, cyclosporine.
   Dental caries.
4. Cessation of nifedipine and improve dental hygiene.

A 44-year-old man had a five-week history of tight retrosternal chest pain on effort. His BP was 150/90 mmHg, heart rate 70 bpm, heart sounds were normal. His cholesterol was 6.8 mmol/l. The resting ECG was normal. An exercise stress test produced chest pain within two minutes of the Bruce protocol, hypotension and the ECG is shown below. Following sublingual glyceryl trinitrate, the ECG normalised. Urgent coronary angiography is shown.

Two minutes of exercise test

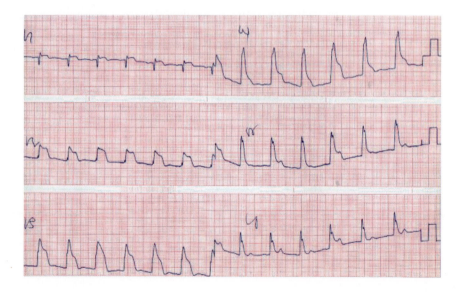

Two minutes post-rest/GTN

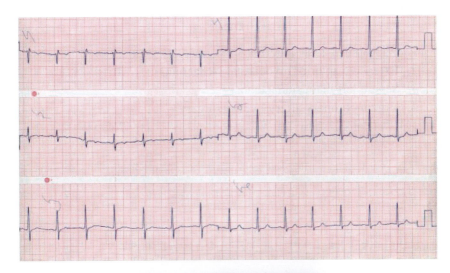

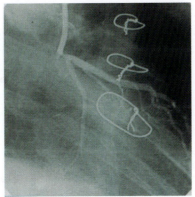

Q Questions:

1. What does the first ECG show?
2. What does it suggest?
3. What does the coronary angiogram show?
4. What treatment is indicated?

Answers:

1. Widespread acute anterior ST-segment elevation.
2. Extensive anterior myocardial ischaemia.
3. Severe left main stem stenosis.
4. Urgent coronary artery bypass surgery.

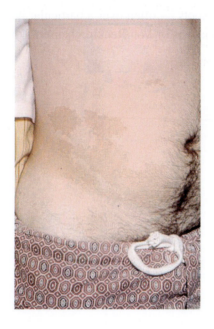

Questions:

1. What is this skin lesion called?
2. With what condition is it usually associated?

Answers:

1. Café-au-lait spots — often over a particular dermatome.
2. Neurofibromatosis or Von Recklinghausen's disease.

A 61-year-old man presented with increased shortness of breath and difficulty in fastening his shirt collar.

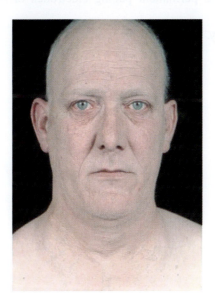

Questions:

1. What two important clinical signs are shown?
2. What is the diagnosis?
3. Name two causes for this condition.
4. What is the first investigation that you would organise? What is the second?

Answers:

1. Swelling of the neck/face and distension of the jugular veins.
2. Superior vena cava obstruction.
3. The commonest cause is bronchogenic carcinoma. Other causes include mediastinal tumours such as lymphoma and thrombosis complicating permanent pacing electrodes or indwelling venous catheters.
4. Chest X-ray. CT scan of thorax.

A *young Asian girl is investigated for persistent anaemia. Her abdomen was distended and there was moderate splenomegaly. The haemoglobin was 6.2 g/100 ml; reticulocyte count 4%. The peripheral blood film is shown.*

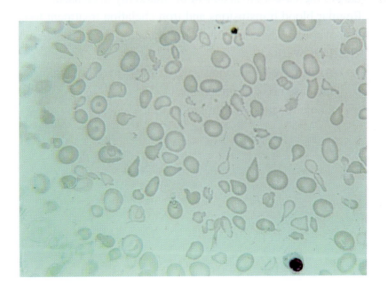

Questions:

1. Name four features seen in the film.
2. What is the diagnosis?
3. What test would you do to confirm the diagnosis?
4. What is the treatment?
5. Give three complications associated with this condition.

Answers:

1. Hypochromia, microcytosis, anisocytosis, poikilocytosis, target cells and nucleated red cell.
2. Thalassaemia major. β-thalassaemia is found in the Far East, parts of India, Burma and Pakistan and is not confined to the Mediterranean.
3. Haemoglobin electrophoresis — Hb F is the major haemoglobin, Hb A2 increased, Hb A absent or markedly decreased.
4. Regular blood transfusions and iron chelation treatment to prevent iron overload. The commonest iron chelating agent is desferoxamine.
5. (i) Iron overload.
   (ii) Asplenia — following splenectomy, may be associated with increased risk of infections.
   (iii) Cholelithiasis — bilirubin stones.

A 70-year-old man complained of breathlessness on effort. He had enjoyed good health until the past three years. He had a cough which was mostly non-productive. He denied haemoptysis, orthopnoea and nocturnal dyspnoea. There was no significant past medical history. He worked as a plumber for most of his life after leaving the "pit". He had spent five years in the local colliery from the age of 16 years.

Physical examination showed mild central cyanosis and finger clubbing. Auscultation of the lung fields revealed fine crepitations bilaterally. The chest X-ray is shown.

Echocardiography showed good left ventricular function.

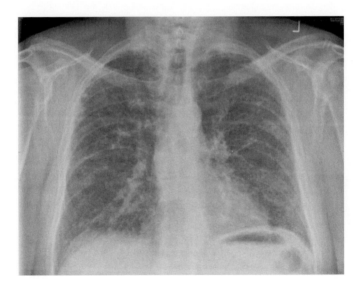

Questions:

1. What does the chest X-ray show?
2. What is the likely diagnosis? What are possible aetiologies?
3. What tests are indicated and what are they likely to show?
4. What treatment can be offered and what is the prognosis?

Answers:

1. Fine reticular/reticulonodular shadowing throughout both lung fields with "honeycombing" — best seen in the apices.

2. Cryptogenic fibrosing alveolitis or idiopathic interstitial pulmonary fibrosis. Asbestosis, sarcoidosis and collagen vascular disorders are possible causes, but seem unlikely here.

3. Pulmonary function testing including lung volume studies and estimation of diffusing capacity. Reduction in total lung capacity, vital capacity and residual volume are likely and the carbon monoxide diffusing capacity may be reduced by 30–50%. High resolution CT scan of lungs may show curvilinear strands coalescing into nodular infiltrates, linear opacities and "honey-combing" of the lung. Fibreoptic bronchoscopy and transbronchial lung biopsies might provide a definitive pathologic diagnosis in 25% of cases. If the biopsies are inadequate for diagnosis, a thoracoscopic-guided or open lung biopsy should be considered before immunosuppressive therapy is entertained.

4. Prednisolone is usually offered to such patients — continued for 6–8 weeks. If no improvement in lung function is demonstrable, addition of cyclophosphamide or azathioprine should be considered. Early involvement of a specialist respiratory physician is paramount.

This elderly gentleman complains of a painful rash affecting his left arm (shown).

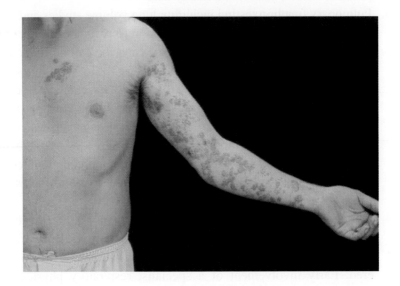

Questions:

1. Describe two important characteristic features of this rash.
2. What is the diagnosis and what is this due to?
3. What are the two commonest complications of this condition in this patient?
4. How would you treat this patient?

Answers:

1. Vesicular rash on an erythematous base, unilateral and along one or two dermatomes. Rash is distributed along T1 dermatome in the picture.
2. Herpes zoster due to reactivation of the varicella-zoster virus.
3. The two commonest complications are secondary bacterial infection of the skin lesions and postherpetic neuralgia.
4. Oral acyclovir or famciclovir. Calamine lotion dabbed onto the vesicles helps them to dry-up. Aluminium acetate dressings might also be soothing and dry the lesions.

This 5-year-old child presents with fever (38.3°C), earache and malaise.

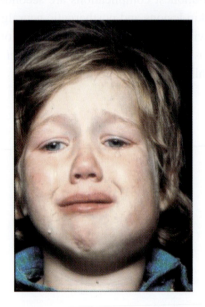

Questions:

1. What one important feature is seen in the picture?
2. What is the diagnosis and name the underlying cause?
3. Name two complications of this condition.

Answers:

1. There is bilateral swelling of the parotid glands in an irritable child.
2. The diagnosis is mumps due to infection with a paramyxovirus.
3. Complications of mumps include aseptic meningitis, encephalitis, transient deafness and orchitis.

Case **38**

A 47-year-old man presented with acute shortness of breath. Physical examination revealed a loud murmur over the precordium and clinical features of pulmonary oedema.

He underwent cardiac catheterisation and the relevant recordings are shown.

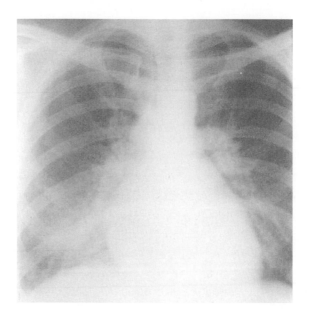

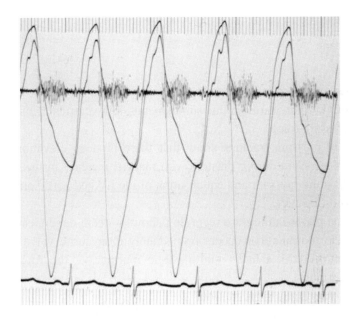

Q Questions:

1. What does the chest X-ray show?
2. What information is being provided on the tracing shown?
3. What does the haemodynamic data show?
4. Describe the type of murmur that is audible.
5. What is the diagnosis?
6. Name two causes for this condition.

Answers:

1. Enlarged cardiac silhouette, pulmonary oedema.
2. ECG, Phonocardiogram, simultaneous left ventricular and aortic pressure traces.
3. The pressure tracings show that there is steep elevation in the LV pressure during diastole with marked increase in the LV end-diastolic pressure and equalisation of the LV and aortic pressure at end-diastole.
4. The phonocardiogram recording shows a decrescendo, early diastolic murmur that occurs immediately after aortic valve closure, followed by a harsh mid-diastolic murmur — the Austin Flint murmur.
5. Severe aortic regurgitation.
6. Acute causes of aortic regurgitation include destruction of the aortic valve due to acute infective endocarditis and acute aortic dissection.

This 50-year-old lady presented with fever, backache, severe headache and photophobia. Examination of the fundi revealed the following appearance.

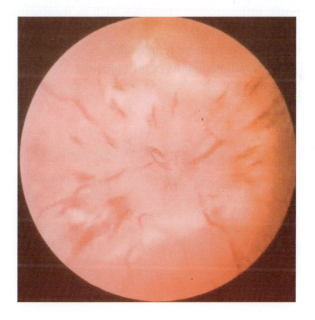

Questions:

1. What is the diagnosis?
2. Name four possible causes.
3. What diagnosis is the most likely?

Answers:

1. The diagnosis is papilloedema. There is gross swelling of the optic disc with peripapillary haemorrhages, exudates and venous congestion.
2.   (i) Any tumours or space-occupying lesions within the skull.
    (ii) Idiopathic intracranial hypertension.
    (iii) Decreased cerebrospinal resorption (e.g. venous sinus thrombosis, inflammatory processes such as meningitis, subarachnoid haemorrhage).
    (iv) Grade 4 hypertensive retinopathy.
3. Viral or bacterial meningitis or encephalitis.

Case 40

A 30-year-old civil engineer returned from Nigeria feeling generally unwell, with headache, fever, tachycardia and soreness and stiffness of his neck. He was concerned about three indurated insect bites — two on his legs and one on his shoulder, which had been very itchy and had become ulcerated. The areas had started to heal and he had been applying an antiseptic cream. Physical examination revealed a temperature of 38.1°C, firm, moderately enlarged lymph nodes in his axillary and inguinal regions and on the back of his neck and mild splenomegaly. He had taken prophylactic antimalarial medication. The ESR was 145 mm in first hour, the white cell count was 12 000/μL and the blood film prepared and stained with a view to establishing the presence of malarial parasites is shown below.

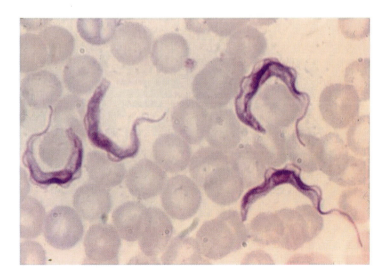

Questions:

1. Describe the appearance of the peripheral blood film.
2. What is the diagnosis?
3. What class of microorganism does it belong to?
4. What is the lay term for this condition?
5. How is it transmitted to man?
6. What treatment should be given?

Answers:

1. The film shows slender, flagellate trypanosomes of up to 30 microns in length with finely pointed anterior and blunted posterior ends, an oval centrally-placed nucleus and a pin-point sized posterior-placed kinetoplast, from which the undulating membrane projects to reach the anterior end of the organism as a free flagellum.
2. African Trypanosomiasis due to *Trypanosoma gambiense*.
3. Protozoa.
4. Sleeping sickness.
5. By the bite of *Glossina* or "tsetse fly".
6. IV pentamidine or Eflornithine (for *T. gambiense*). IV suramin for *T. rhodesiense*.

> *This is an ECG trace from an 18-year-old patient with palpitations.*

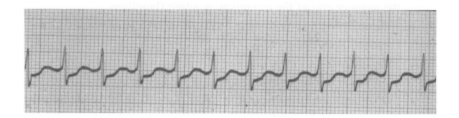

Questions:

1. What is the diagnosis and heart rate?
2. What treatment would you give?
3. Name two underlying electrophysiological causes for the arrhythmia.

Answers:

1. The diagnosis is supraventricular tachycardia and the heart rate is 180 bpm.
2. Intravenous adenosine causing temporary atrioventricular block. This would terminate a tachycardia that uses the AV node as part of its pathway.
3. The absence of visible P waves and a regular rate suggests either atrioventricular re-entrant tachycardia (AVRT) or atrioventricular nodal re-entrant tachycardia (AVNRT).

   AVRT is due to an accessory pathway that conducts retrogradely during the tachycardia with antegrade conduction down the AV node. The ECG in sinus rhythm may show pre-excitation in a patient with Wolff–Parkinson–White syndrome or no changes in the presence of a concealed accessory pathway (one that does not conduct anterogradely during sinus rhythm).

   AVNRT is due to a re-entry pathway within the AV node itself.

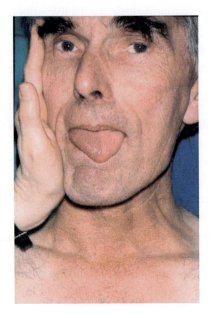

uestions:

1. What neurological abnormality is being demonstrated here?
2. What is the likely diagnosis?

Answers:

1. A left 12th cranial nerve palsy with a wasted left half of tongue, deviation of the tongue to the left on protrusion. A left 11th cranial nerve palsy with a weak left sternomastoid.
2. Motor neurone disease.

A 74-year-old man presented with cough and dyspnoea with severe upper back pain radiating around to the front of his chest. He had hypertension for six years, treated with amlodipine and lisinopril. He smoked 15 cigarettes per day. His ECG was normal. The chest-X-ray is shown.

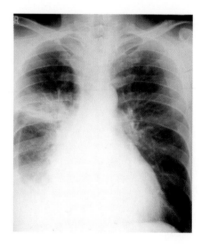

Questions:

1. Name three abnormal features on the chest X-ray.
2. What is the most likely diagnosis?
3. What investigation would you do first?
4. What two investigations would you do next?
5. What is the likely cause of his back pain and what two tests would you request to try and elucidate the cause?

Answers:

1. There is a large right pleural effusion, abnormal right hilum and area of consolidation affecting the right mid-zone.
2. Bronchogenic carcinoma.
3. Computed tomography of the chest.
4. Pleural aspiration for cytology and microbiology. Bronchoscopy.
5. Metastatic deposits in the upper thoracic vertebra(e) with possible wedge collapse. X-ray of thoracic spine (PA and lateral) and bone scan.

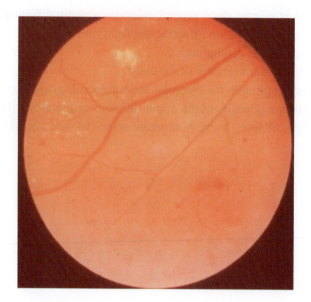

Questions:

1. Name three abnormalities in this fundus.
2. What is the diagnosis?

Answers:

1. Hard exudates; dot microaneurysms/haemorrhages; blot haemorrhages, arteriolar narrowing.
2. Diabetes mellitus retinopathy.

A 70-year-old man with a history of previous coronary artery bypass surgery and a prostatectomy presented with severe pain in the left shoulder and pleuritic pain in the right side of his chest. Routine blood count showed haemoglobin 10.1 g/dL; white cell count 2 500/μL; platelets 90 000/μL. The peripheral blood film (top) and the bone marrow aspirate (bottom) are shown.

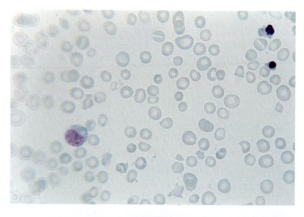

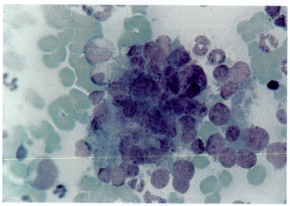

Questions:

1. What is the diagnosis from the blood count?
2. What does the peripheral blood film show?
3. What does the bone marrow show?
4. What is the likely diagnosis?
5. What is the cause of his chest and shoulder pain?
6. What other tests are required?
7. What are other causes of this complication?

Answers:

1. Pancytopaenia.
2. Leucoerythroblastic anaemia.
3. The aspirate shows darkly stained clumps of malignant cells in the bone marrow, suggesting bone metastases.
4. Bony metastases from adenocarcinoma of the prostate.
5. Rib, clavicular, humeral or scapular deposits.
6. Serum prostate specific antigen, radioisotope bone scan.
7. Common cancers that metastasise to bone including lung, breast, thyroid, kidney, as well as prostate.

This 66-year-old ex-seafarer complained of dull, substernal pain. His symptoms occurred both at rest and on effort, especially at night. More recently, he had noticed a persistent cough and some hoarseness of his voice. He smoked 20 cigarettes per day. Physical examination revealed an ejection systolic murmur over the aortic area and an early diastolic murmur at the left sternal edge. The ECG showed sinus rhythm, left ventricular hypertrophy, ST depression and T-wave inversion in leads V5-6, leads I and AVL. The chest X-ray is shown.

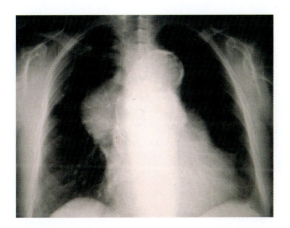

Questions:

1. What does the chest X-ray show?
2. What is the likely diagnosis?
3. What three tests are indicated?
4. What treatment should be offered?

A̶nswers:

1. Cardiac enlargement, aneurysmal dilatation of the ascending aorta, thin, linear calcification of the ascending aorta extending down into the root.
2. Syphilitic aortitis and aortic regurgitation.
3. Serology (TPHA, FTA-abs), echocardiography, cardiac catheterisation, including aortography and coronary arteriography.
4. Aortic root and valve replacement, possibly with concomitant coronary artery bypass surgery.

A 58-year-old man presented with a three-month history of malaise, night sweats and weight loss of one stone. He complained of severe left upper quadrant abdominal pain. The appearance of his fingers is shown below. His temperature was 38.2°C; BP 160/80 mmHg; pulse rate 108 bpm. A mid-systolic click and late systolic murmur was audible with radiation to the left axilla. There was severe tenderness and guarding over the left hypochondrium. Routine urine testing showed erythrocytes and leucocytes. Haemoglobin 10.3 g/dL; white cell count 15 000/μL, C-reactive protein 150 mg/dL.

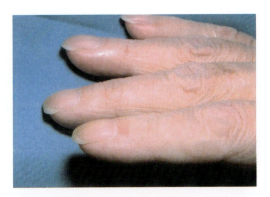

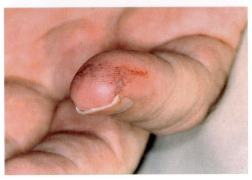

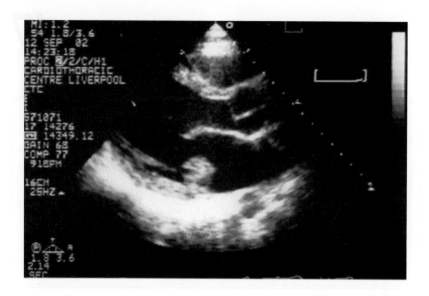

Questions:

1. What single question should be asked?
2. What investigation is shown? What is demonstrated by the investigation?
3. What other tests are of paramount importance?
4. What is the likely diagnosis? What treatment is necessary?

Answers:

1. Has he received any dental or surgical treatment recently and did he have antibiotic prophylaxis? He had had a "wisdom tooth" removed without antibiotic cover three and one half months earlier. His parents had previously been told that he had a heart murmur but no investigations were done. His undiagnosed mitral valve prolapse/mitral regurgitation had caused no symptoms. The pictures show early finger clubbing and an Osler's node at the tip of the thumb.

2. 2-D echocardiography. Large spherical vegetation is present on the posterior leaflet of the mitral valve.

3. Blood cultures, CT scan of the abdomen.

4. Infective endocarditis, with vegetation on a prolapsing mitral valve. Splenic infarction. Treatment should be commenced with intravenous antibiotics — dose and type of antibiotics dependent on results of blood cultures. Cardiac surgery may be required to replace the infected mitral valve.

Case **48**

This 52-year-old aid worker became ill whist working in a refugee camp in Ethiopia. He felt generally unwell for two days before developing headache, widespread aches and pains, nausea and vomiting, rigors and a patchy erythematous rash on his limbs and trunk. His temperature rose rapidly to 40°C and continued as a remittent fever. His conjunctivae were injected and he had blood stained discharge from his nose. Within four days he became jaundiced and physical examination revealed tender hepato-splenomegaly. He attended a local hospital where it was noticed that his clothes were infested with lice and his skin was covered in excoriations. Following a collapse, he was resuscitated with IV fluids and his temperature abated. Three days later, however, the pyrexia and rigors returned. Blood was taken during a febrile period. He had a leucocytosis and the Giemsa-stained blood film is shown.

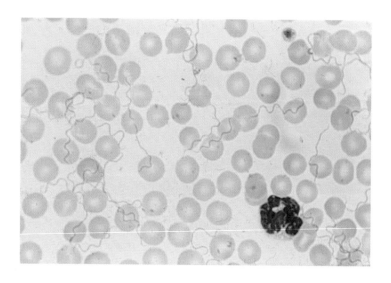

Questions:

1. What does the peripheral blood film show?
2. What is the likely diagnosis?
3. How can the diagnosis be confirmed?
4. What treatment is necessary?

Answers:

1. Spirochaetes are seen in the blood film preparation.
2. Relapsing fever due to *Borrelia recurrentis* infection.
3. Although the history, the presence of lice and the blood film make the diagnosis likely, an immunofluorescence assay (IFA) and an enzyme-linked immunosorbent assay (ELISA) have been shown to identify antibodies to Glycerophosphodiester Phosphodiesterase (GlpQ) i.e. anti-GlpQ antibodies, from *Borrelia recurrentis.* However, such assays will probably only be available in special microbiology laboratories.
4. The louse infestation must be removed and the patient treated with DDT and bathed on admission. Tetracycline 500 mg qds for one day, followed by 250 mg qds for one week. The course is repeated after one week.

A 53-year-old man gave a six-month history of progressive dyspnoea and a four month history of increasing abdominal distension, nausea and anorexia. He complained of worsening fatigue, lethargy and mild ankle swelling. On examination, he was apyrexial; jugular venous pressure markedly elevated; heart rate 90 bpm; BP 105/70 mmHg. There was reduced air entry at the right base, quiet heart sounds and a third heart sound was audible at the left sternal edge. There was marked ascites but no significant peripheral oedema.

The ECG showed sinus rhythm. The chest X-ray showed a normal heart size but a modest sized right basal pleural effusion. The lateral chest X-ray, ECG and the haemodynamic data at cardiac catheterisation are shown.

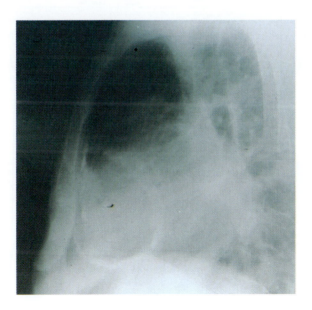

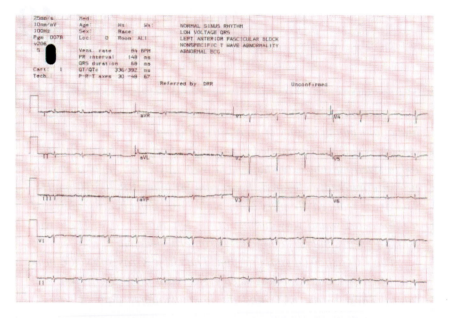

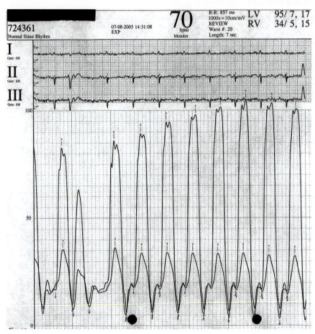

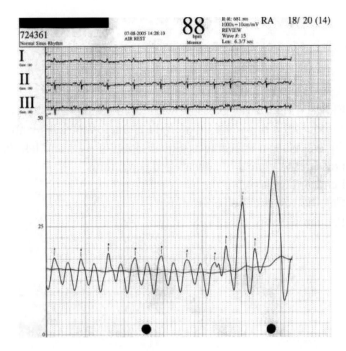

Questions:

1. What does the chest X-ray show?
2. What does the catheter data show?
3. What other investigation might have been helpful?
4. What is the diagnosis?
5. What treatment is required?

Answers:

1. A ring of calcification surrounding the heart.
2. Elevated right atrial pressure with rapid X and Y descents; raised end diastolic pressures in the right and left ventricles with typical dip and plateau appearance. Equalisation of right and left diastolic pressures is typical of constrictive pericarditis.
3. Echocardiography.
4. Calcific constrictive pericarditis.
5. Pericardiectomy.

Case **50**

This 5-year-old child had a swelling in the neck.

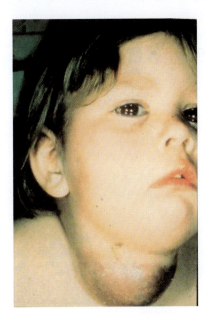

Q Questions:

1. What is the diagnosis?
2. What treatment is indicated?

Answers:

1. Thyroglossal cyst.
2. Surgical removal.

A 76-year-old man with maturity onset diabetes mellitus, hypercholesterolaemia, hypertension and a history of coronary artery bypass surgery was well until his home in Florida was devastated by a hurricane. He received numerous insect bites whilst searching amongst the ruins. Within 48 hours, he became unwell, with fatigue, lethargy, myalgia, rigors and anorexia. Despite deteriorating, he did not seek medical attention until returning to the UK three weeks later by which time he had lost two stones in weight. He received oral cephalosporin but this was not based on evidence of infection or the result of any investigation. On examination, he looked unwell with a sallow complexion. He was initially apyrexial. Abdominal examination revealed fullness and tenderness in the left hypochondrium but no palpable mass. Investigations showed leucocytosis 19 000/μL — 95% neutrophils. C-reactive protein (CRP) was 160 mg/dL. Abdominal ultrasound confirmed splenomegaly with a suggestion of an echolucent area within the spleen. The CT scan of the abdomen is shown.

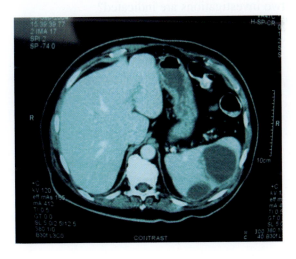

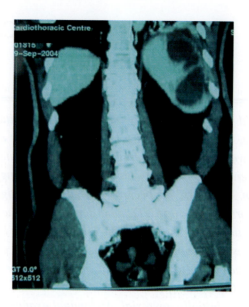

Questions:

1. What does the CT scan show?
2. What is the likely diagnosis?
3. What two investigations are indicated?
4. What treatment is necessary?

Answers:

1. A large multilobulated, low density mass within the spleen extending close to the capsular surface.
2. Splenic abscess.
3. Blood cultures — *Escherichia coli* was grown; microbiological culture and sensitivity of fluid removed from the splenic abscess.
4. Percutaneous drainage of the splenic abscess. Intravenous antibiotics to include agents active against gram-positive, gram-negative and anaerobic organisms until the results of the microbiology tests are available. *E. coli* was grown from the 500 mls of thick chocolate-brown pus aspirated from the abscess cavity and IV ceftriaxone, gentamicin and metronidazole was given.
   Antibiotics were instilled into the abscess cavity.

A 58-year-old woman with congestive cardiac failure due to rheumatic mitral and aortic valve disease presented with severe dyspnoea and leg oedema. Although she responded well to medical treatment, nine days after commencing therapy, she developed itchy painful rash on her arms and legs. The eruption is shown below.

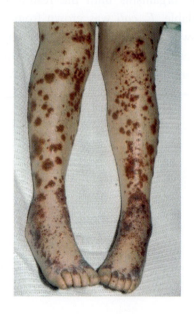

Q Questions:

1. Describe the rash.
2. What is the likely cause?
3. What should be done?

Answers:

1. Symmetrical, orange-brown papulo-vesicular eruption with associated purpura and haemorrhagic blisters.
2. Drug-induced vasculitis — almost certainly due to frusemide.
3. Stop the frusemide and change to bumetanide.

Case **53**

A 49-year-old man was referred to the rheumatologist because of severe back and joint pains. The knee and ankle joints were mainly affected. He was troubled by severe morning stiffness lasting for 3–4 hours each day. Over the past 18 months he had noticed dry, "gritty" eyes and large aphthous ulcers in his mouth and in the past four weeks had noticed burning discomfort at the distal end of his penis on passing urine, superficial ulcers on the glans penis and pale yellow urethral discharge. The following were found on physical examination: BP 150/65 mmHg; heart rate 100 bpm; short early diastolic murmur at the left sternal edge and crepitations over the lung fields. Both knee and ankle joints were swollen and tender to pressure. The penis is shown below. The ESR was 120 mm in the first hour, white cell count 12 500/μL.

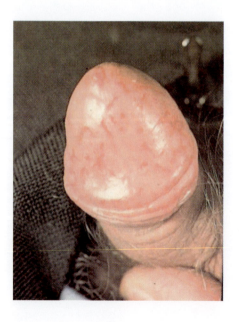

Questions:

1. What is the likely diagnosis?
2. What does the picture show?
3. What investigations are required?
4. What is the cause of his urinary symptoms?
5. What treatment should he be offered?

Answers:

1. Reiter's syndrome.
2. Circinate balanitis or superficial ulceration on the glans penis.
3. Microscopy, culture and sensitivity of urethral discharge to exclude gonococcal infection; rheumatoid factor; opthalmological examination to distinguish between conjunctivitis, uveitis and keratitis.
4. Urethritis (non-specific) is a feature of Reiter's syndrome.
5. Rest and aspirin or non-steroidal anti-inflammatory drug for the arthritis, light splints at night might help. A dilute hydrocortisone cream might help circinate balanitis. Tetracycline 250–500 mg qds for 5–20 days might help urethritis. Systemic steroid therapy may be necessary for severe arthritis or anterior uveitis.

A 25-year-old woman complained of breathlessness, which was diagnosed as asthma by her general practitioner. She was referred to a chest physician for advice. The chest X-ray is shown.

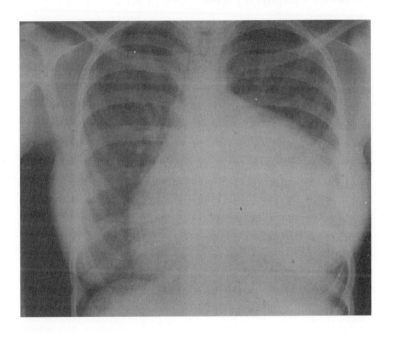

Questions:

1. What does the chest X-ray show?
2. What are the three possible causes?
3. What are the two most useful investigations?

Answers:

1. Massive cardiac silhouette.
2 (i) Large pericardial effusion;
   (ii) Thymoma;
   (iii) Dilated cardiac chambers e.g. left atrium, right atrium, right
        and left ventricles.
3 Echocardiography; CT scan.

This irritating lesion on the face of this patient had enlarged progressively over the last seven months.

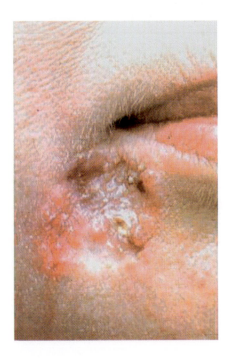

Questions:

1. What is this skin lesion?
2. What treatment is indicated?

Answers:

1. Basal cell carcinoma.
2. Radiotherapy/plastic surgery.

Case **56**

A 23-year-old Indian man was visiting relatives in the UK when he complained of pain and swelling in the scrotum and tender, swollen glands in the left inguinal region. He had experienced similar symptoms previously at home. He found that walking caused pain in the region of the left hip and thigh. He felt generally unwell and was off his food. He had noticed intermittent fever and shivering episodes. On examination, he was pyrexial 37.8°C with cervical, axillary and inguinal lymphadenopathy. The scrotum was slightly swollen and inflamed and the left testis enlarged and exquisitely tender. There was a moderate sized hydrocoele. The top of his thigh was oedematous and there was streaky erythema. The area was tender to touch and very itchy and excoriations from scratching were visible. The left inguinal nodes were large and tender.

Investigations revealed haemoglobin 11.6 g/dL; white cell count 18 000/μL with a marked eosinophilia. The stained thick film was made from venous blood taken during a febrile episode.

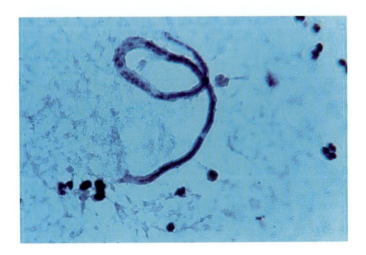

Questions:

1. What does the image show?
2. What is the diagnosis?
3. What is the cause of the physical signs?
4. What treatment is necessary?
5. What should be of concern after initiating treatment?

Answers:

1. Microfilaria is seen in this thick blood film preparation after filtering haemolysed blood (with dilute tepol) through a millipore filter.
2. *Wuchereria bancrofti* filariasis.
3. Severe inguinal lymphadenitis, local oedema and lymphangitis of the skin, funiculitis and orchitis.
4. Diethylcarbamazepine.
5. Acute allergic reactions in the first few days of treatment since it rapidly kills off the microfilariae. These may include acute oedema, often involving face and neck, remittent fever, local oedema and urticaria.

Case 57

A 9-year-old boy from Uganda was visiting his relatives in Liverpool when he developed left hypochondrial pain and dark-coloured urine. He appeared mildly icteric and the spleen was palpable. His blood count revealed haemoglobin 7.0 g/dL; white cell count 8 200/μL. The peripheral blood film is shown.

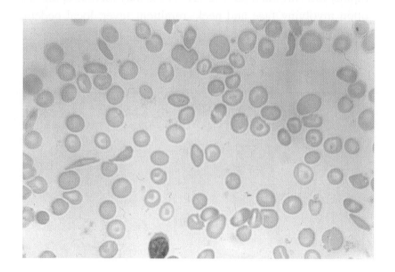

Questions:

1. Give four abnormalities seen on the blood film.
2. What is the diagnosis?
3. What tests might confirm the diagnosis?

Answers:

1. Anisocytosis, sickle cells, elliptocytes, target cells, red cells containing Howell–Jolly bodies, fragmented and crenated erythrocytes.
2. Sickle-cell anaemia.
3. Haemoglobin electrophoresis shows haemoglobin S with an elevation of foetal haemoglobin of 5–10%. An elevated reticulocyte count and raised bilirubin. Sickling can be demonstrated by incubating the cells in sodium metabisulphite under a coverslip sealed by Vaseline.

A 20-year-old female developed palpitations when dancing in a nightclub. Although the "fluttering sensations" were initially brief, they became sustained. Her friends became concerned and called for an ambulance. Within a few minutes of the ambulance arriving, she felt faint and breathless with tightness in her chest. The paramedics recorded the ECG shown and took her quickly to a heart emergency centre for treatment. After successful treatment, the second ECG was recorded.

FIRST ECG

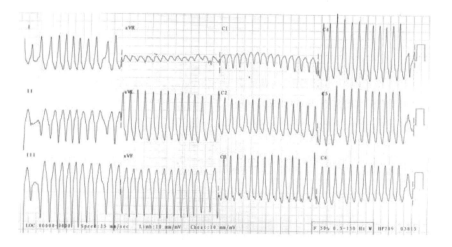

SECOND ECG

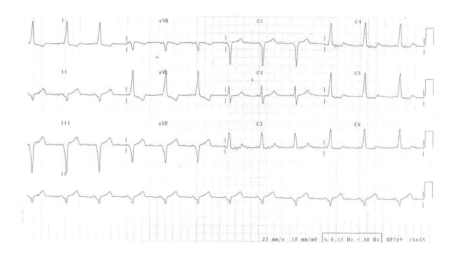

Questions:

1. What rhythm disturbance is evident in the first ECG?
2. Why was she so symptomatic?
3. What treatment should be given?
4. What does the second ECG show?
5. What is the diagnosis? What definitive investigation and treatment could be offered?

Answers:

1. Rapid atrial fibrillation with pre-excitation.
2. Low cardiac output causing hypotension as a result of a ventricular rate of almost 300 bpm.
3. IV flecainide in the absence of severe hypotension (if systolic BP ≥ 100 mmHg) or DC Cardioversion.
4. After a successful DC Cardioversion, the 12 lead ECG shows Wolff–Parkinson–White syndrome Type B, with visible δ-wave, short PR interval and wide QRS complex.
5. Wolff–Parkinson–White syndrome, Type B. Electrophysiological study with view to identification of the accessory pathway and its ablation by radio frequency.

This 35-year-old homosexual man returned from vacation in Tunisia feeling unwell, with remittent fever, sweating and with bloody diarrhoea. He had discomfort in the right hypochondrium. On examination, he had a temperature of 37.5°C, mild tender hepatomegaly and generalised tenderness over the abdomen. His white cell count was 12 500/μL and the ESR 50 mm in first hour. Stools were sent for microscopy, culture and sensitivity testing. Microscopy of the faecal smear is shown after iodine staining.

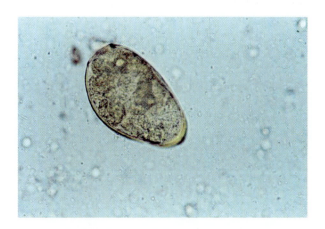

Questions:

1. What does the picture show?
2. What is the diagnosis?
3. What treatment should he be given?
4. How has the infection been acquired?

Answers:

1. The trophozoite of *Entamoeba histolytica.*
2. Intestinal amoebiasis or amoebic dysentery.
3. Metronidazole 800 mg tds for 7–10 days.
4. Probably by ingestion of drinking water or food infected by the cysts of the parasite. Infection can also occur as a result of homosexual activity due to oro-anal and oro-genital contact.

A 71-year-old man was referred because of breathlessness nine years after undergoing coronary artery bypass surgery. He also had angina of effort and was limited to < 100 yards of physical effort because of both symptoms. He was on atenolol 50 mg/day, aspirin 75 mg/day, simvastatin 20 mg/day. On examination he was over-weight, BP 160/95 mmHg, heart rate 75 bpm, heart sounds normal. Abdominal examination revealed gross splenomegaly. The haemoglobin was 7.1 g/dL, white cell count 12 000/μL, platelets 90 000/μL. ESR 40 mm in the first hour, CRP 96 mg/dL. The chest X-ray showed cardiomegaly but clear lung fields. Faecal occult bloods were negative. A bone marrow aspirate was attempted but failed. A bone marrow trephine from the iliac crest is shown.

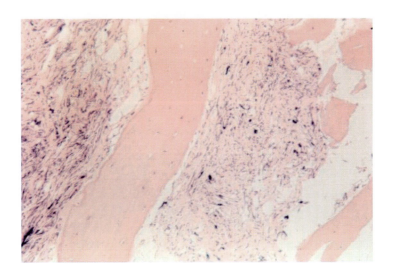

Questions:

1. What does the picture show?
2. What is the diagnosis?
3. What treatment should be offered?

Answers:

1. Between the bony trabeculae is dense fibrous tissue, densely-stained nuclei of varying sizes and multinucleated cells. Absence of bone marrow.
2. Myelofibrosis. The splenomegaly is thought to be due to extramedullary erythropoesis because of myeloid metaplasia.
3. Blood transfusion.

Case **61**

> This 45-year-old man is on an intensive care unit requiring naso-gastric feeding and hydration.

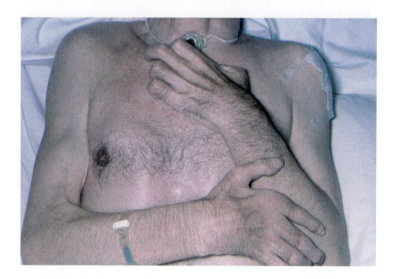

Questions:

1. What three features are evident in the illustration?
2. What are the two possible causes?

Answers:

1. Tracheostomy; muscle wasting in the upper limbs; wasting of the small muscles of the hands and "main en griffe" appearance of the hands.
2. Motor neurone disease; cervical cord injury.

This 50-year-old man complained of a bleeding ulcer on his scrotum. It had appeared as a small papule which seemed to enlarge fairly quickly before eroding as shown.

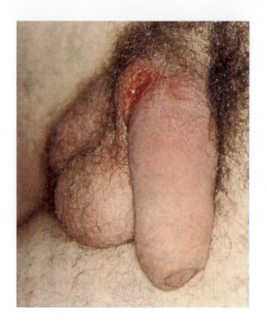

Questions:

1. What is the likely diagnosis?
2. What three tests should be done?
3. What treatment is indicated?

Answers:

1. Primary syphilitic chancre due to *Treponema pallidum*.
2. Microscopy of exudates from ulcer for spirochaetes; Fluorescent Treponemal Antibody (FTA) test; *Treponema pallidum* Immobilization (TPI) test.
3. IM penicillin — 10–12 daily IM injections of 1G of procaine penicillin.

Case 63

A 42-year-old man complained of sore, red eyes and of feeling gen-erally fatigued and lethargic and a poor appetite. He had lost one stone in weight over the past six months and for the past 12 months had had recurrent ulcers in his mouth and on his tongue. He had noticed a rash on his forearm and a painful lesion on his scrotum.

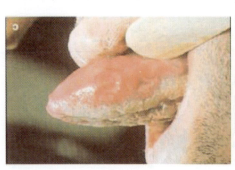 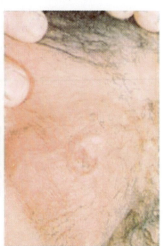

Questions:

1. What is the likely diagnosis?
2. What is the cause of his sore eyes?
3. What test might confirm it?
4. What treatment could be offered?
5. What other complications may occur?

Answers:

1. Behçet's syndrome.
2. Conjunctivitis, iridocyclitis and uveitis are typical ocular lesions that might occur.
3. There are no specific diagnostic tests. The triad of iritis, recurrent buccal and genital ulcers make the diagnosis likely.
4. Corticosteroids will suppress the acute inflammatory episodes and long term steroids might keep the condition under control.
5. Recurrent epididymitis, pericarditis, thrombosis of large veins and central nervous system involvement such as a "brain stem syndrome", a meningomyelitis or an organic confusional state.

Case **64**

A 36-year-old electrician had noticed effort-related chest pain and breathlessness over the past six months, but he went to his general practitioner because he had collapsed on the squash court after several episodes of feeling lightheaded. There was no significant past medical history. He was on no medication and was a non-smoker. Physical examination revealed heart rate 75 bpm; BP 140/80 mmHg and an ejection systolic murmur at the left sternal edge and over the 2nd right intercostal space. The murmur radiated into the neck and the carotid pulse appeared to have a sharp upstroke.

The important investigations are shown below.

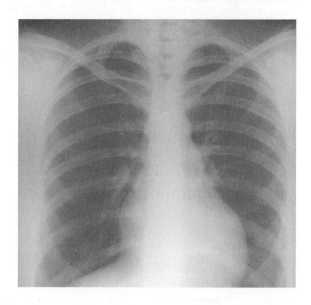

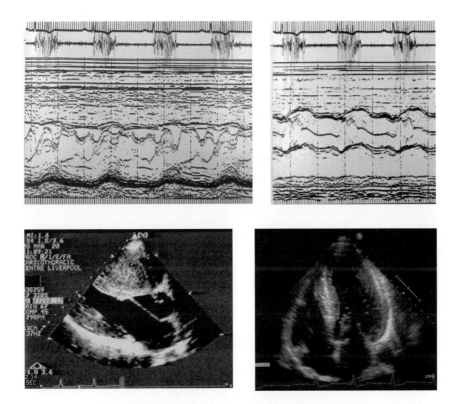

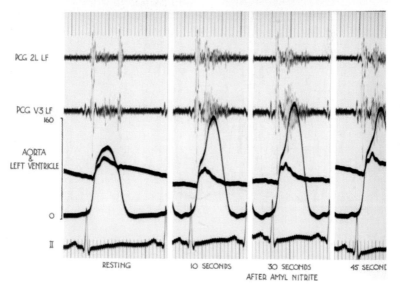

RESTING   IO SECONDS   3O SECONDS   45 SECOND

AFTER AMYL NITRITE

Questions:

1. What three investigations are shown?
2. What do the investigations show?
3. What is the diagnosis?
4. What is the first line treatment?
5. What are the other two treatment options?

Answers:

1. PA chest X-ray; echocardiogram; cardiac catheterisation with simultaneous LV and aortic pressures before and after amyl nitrite.
2. Chest X-ray: LV enlargement.
   Echocardiogram: Asymmetric septal hypertrophy, systolic anterior motion of the mitral valve; left ventricular hypertrophy; premature closure of the aortic valve.
   Left ventricular outflow tract gradient increases markedly after inhalation of amyl nitrite confirms the diagnosis.
3. Hypertrophic obstructive cardiomyopathy.
4. β-blocker e.g. atenolol, sotalol, propranolol.
5. Percutaneous alcohol septal ablation or septal myectomy.

A 67-year-old man presented with chest pain due to acute anterior myocardial infarction two weeks after implantation of a bare-metal stent to his left anterior descending coronary artery. He was treated with IV tenecteplase and transferred for emergency coronary angiography and possibly percutaneous coronary intervention (PCI). The LAD was patent but there was visible thrombus in the diagonal coronary artery. He was given intracoronary abciximab and there was rapid improvement. However, 24 hours later he developed further chest pain and ST-elevation and was found to have acute LAD occlusion at the proximal end of the stent (shown). He was given 8000 U of heparin for his emergency PCI and intracoronary bolus of abciximab followed by IV infusion over 12 hours. The LAD was opened by balloon angioplasty and restented with a further two bare metal stents. The angiograms before and after PCI are shown. He was already taking aspirin and clopidogrel following his first PCI. The following day his platelet count was 58 000/μL and 24 hours later was 26 000/μL. He had no spontaneous bleeding.

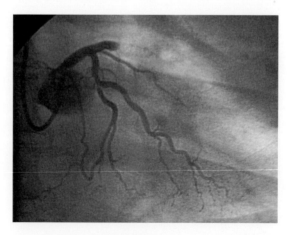

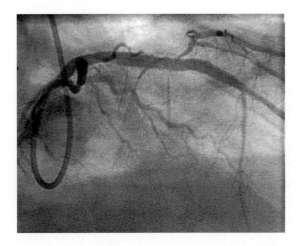

Questions:

1. What is the current problem?
2. What are the possible causes?
3. What investigations are necessary?
4. What treatment is possibly indicated?

Answers:

1. Thrombocytopaenia.
2. Clopidogrel therapy.
   Abciximab therapy.
   Heparin-induced thrombocytopaenia (HIT).
3. Platelet factor 4 antibody titre.
4. If platelet count starts to return to normal within the next 24–48 hours, the thrombocytopaenia is likely to be due to abciximab. PF4 antibodies were not detected and so HIT is unlikely. For HIT, IV hirudin or IV/sc Danaparoid is indicated. If the platelet count fails to rise or continues to fall, the clopidogrel would be discontinued and IV Danaparoid 750 U sc bd given for four weeks.

A 77-year-old man complained of breathlessness on minimal effort over the past five years. He had smoked 30 cigarettes per day since he was 23 years of age. He worked as a bookbinder for most of his working life. He was receiving no treatment. The chest X-ray and pulmonary function tests are shown.

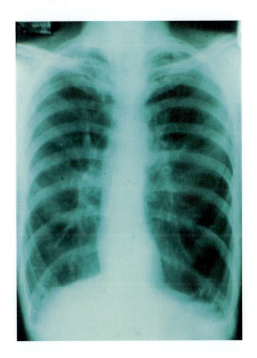

FVC: 2.1 L (pred 5.1 L); FEV1: 1.0 L (pred 4.1 L); PEFR: 4.1 L/sec (pred 9.2 L/sec) FEV1/FVC: 47.6% (pred 80.1%); TLC: 8.1 L (pred 7.2 L); RV: 5.4 L (pred 2.6 L) DLCO: 12.2 mL/min/mmHg (pred 30.4)

Q

Questions:

1. What does the chest X-ray show?
2. What do the pulmonary function tests show?
3. What is the diagnosis?
4. What treatment can be offered?

Answers:

1. Hyperinflated lung fields; low flat diaphragms; small heart shadow.
2. Reduced FVC; reduced FEV1; reduced FEV1/FVC ratio; reduced peak expiratory flow rate; increased total lung capacity; increased residual volume; reduced transfer factor.
3. Emphysema.
4. Bronchodilator therapy e.g. salbutamol, atrovent; domiciliary oxygen.

Case **67**

This 56-year-old homosexual complained of cough and mild breathlessness as well as a diminished appetite and one stone weight loss over the previous month.

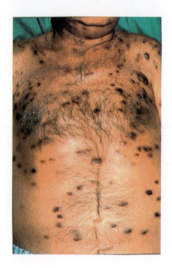

Questions:

1. What does the picture show?
2. What is the diagnosis?
3. What is the cause of his symptoms?
4. What tests are appropriate?
5. What should be particularly considered? What tests might be required if seriously a possibility?
6. What treatment should be offered?

Answers:

1. Purple nodular lesions on skin of thorax and abdomen (also on hands and feet — not seen).
2. Kaposi's sarcoma.
3. Respiratory infection, pulmonary sarcomatous nodules or pleural effusions.
4. Chest X-ray, arterial blood gas analysis, microscopy/culture/sensitivity of sputum, blood count, CD4 count, HIV testing, viral serology, possibly CT scan.
5. *Pneumocystis carinii* infection. Sputum, induced-sputum, fibre-optic bronchoscopy with bronchoalveolar lavage or bronchial biopsies — silver staining for pneumocysts.
6. Chemotherapy/biological response modifiers e.g. γ-interferon/radiotherapy should be considered. If *Pneumocystis carinii* is identified, first-line treatment should be with trimethoprim/sulphamethoxazole (Bactrim, Septrin).

This 73-year-old man complained of pain on the right side of his head and earache.

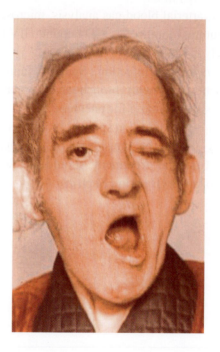

Q Questions:

1. What manoeuvre has he been asked to perform?
2. What three abnormalities can be seen in the picture?
3. What is the pathology?
4. What is the diagnosis?

Answers:

1. He has been asked to close his eyes tightly and screw up his face.
2. Right-sided ptosis; right sided facial palsy; vesicles/calamine lotion on his right ear.
3. Herpes zoster (shingles) affecting the right geniculate ganglion.
4. Ramsay Hunt syndrome.

This 73-year-old man complained of exertional dyspnoea which had become worse over the past three years. He was limited to 150 yards on level ground and was particularly short of breath on inclines. He used three pillows at night. He had no angina but had suffered a myocardial infarction ten years earlier. He had smoked cigarettes for over 50 years and still smoked ten cigarettes per day. The ECG and chest X-ray are shown.

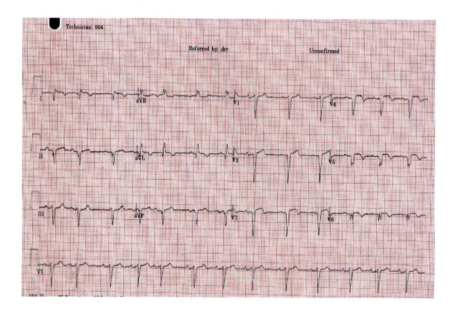

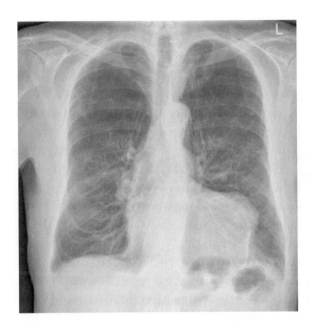

Questions:

1. What two abnormalities are evident on the ECG?
2. What two diagnoses are obvious on the chest X-ray?
3. What two clinical features are likely to be found on physical examination?
4. What three investigations are indicated?
5. What treatment could he be offered?

Answers:

1. (i) Deep Q-waves in leads V1–V6, I, II, aVF.
    (ii) Persistent ST-elevation in leads V1–V6, I and aVL.
2. (i) Bilateral upper lobe emphysema.
    (ii) Cardiomegaly with an abnormal "boot-shaped" contour, due to left ventricular aneurysm.
3. (i) Reduced breath sounds in both upper lobes.
    (ii) Paradoxical apical impulse.
4. (i) Pulmonary function tests.
    (ii) Echocardiography.
    (iii) Cardiac catheterisation including left ventricular angiography.
5. He should stop smoking and if reversibility of airways obstruction is demonstrated by pulmonary function testing, bronchodilator therapy might be helpful. If a large localised left ventricular aneurysm is demonstrated by left ventricular angiography, surgical resection could be considered. He would have to possess reasonable pulmonary function before he could be accepted for open heart surgery.

This young woman with epilepsy had these skin lesions on her back

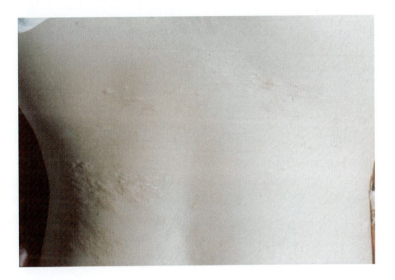

Questions:

1. What is this skin lesion called?
2. What is the diagnosis?

Answers:

1. Shagreen patch — an area of rough, leathery skin, often dimpled and likened to orange peel.
2. Tuberous sclerosis.

Case **71**

This 22-year-old woman complained of intermittent pain and coldness in the fingers of her right hand and shooting pains down her right arm. She worked on an assembly line in a local car components factory. Her symptoms tended to worsen as the day progressed. She was referred to a cardiologist because of intermittent palpitations over the previous six months. Physical examination revealed no abnormalities. Routine investigations revealed haemoglobin 12.1 g/dL; white cell count 8000/μL; platelet count 105 000/μL; ESR 4; Free T4 17 pmol/L; TSH 1.5 mU/L. The chest X-ray is shown.

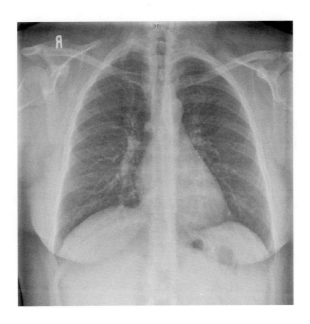

Questions:

1. What is the diagnosis?
2. What is the cause of the symptoms?
3. What simple clinical test can you do to support the diagnosis?
4. What treatment is necessary?

Answers:

1. Cervical rib syndrome.
2. Right cervical rib. Found on 0.4% of chest X-rays and 70% are bilateral. Neurological symptoms are uncommon but pain in the ulnar distribution, aching in the shoulder or scapular region may occur.
3. Adson's deep breathing test depends on the fact that the scalenus anterior is an accessory muscle of respiration. Feel the radial pulse of the seated patient, who is asked to turn the head as far possible *towards* the side of the symptoms. When asked, the patient takes a deep breath, and holds it. If inspiration causes a diminution or obliteration of the pulse, the sign is positive. A subclavian murmur suggests that the artery is angulated over an obstruction.
4. Resection of the cervical rib.

This 76-year-old West Indian man presented with a six month history of increasing exertional dyspnoea and ankle swelling. He had no angina. He had been treated for pulmonary tuberculosis at the age of 19 years. On examination he looked well but the JVP was raised 6 cm, BP 150/85 mmHg, pulse 90/min, he had moderate ankle oedema and there was a soft mid-systolic murmur at the left sternal edge and apex. The ECG showed low voltage complexes and small r-waves in V1–V4. The chest X-ray showed mild cardiomegaly and mild pulmonary venous congestion. The echocardiogram is shown.

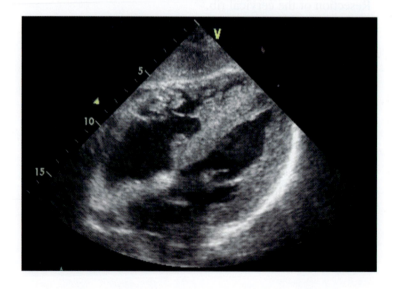

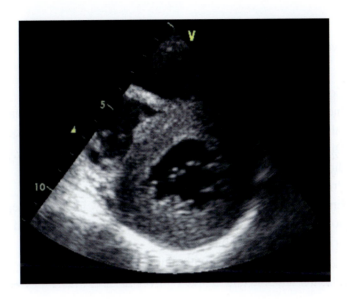

Questions:

1. What is the clinical diagnosis?
2. What does the echocardiogram show?
3. What is the pathophysiological explanation for the clinical findings? How can this be confirmed?
4. What is the likely aetiology?
5. What investigation is necessary to confirm this?
6. What treatment is indicated?
7. What two treatments are probably contraindicated?

Answers:

1. Congestive cardiac failure.
2. Increased thickness of right and left ventricular walls, increased septal thickness, "granular" or "sparkly" appearance to the myocardium.
3. Diastolic dysfunction causing restrictive defect. Doppler echocardiography should confirm impaired diastolic relaxation.
4. Primary cardiac amyloidosis.
5. Endomyocardial biopsy. Histology will show interstitial deposits of homogenous material which stains with Congo Red and appears bright green under polarised light.
6. Symptomatic treatment with diuretics.
7. Digoxin and calcium channel blockers.

Case 73

This 70-year-old man presented with recurrent dizziness and was found to have complete heart block on the ECG. He was also found to have recurrent ventricular tachycardia and an impaired left ventricle. He underwent dual chamber pacemaker/automatic implantable cardioverter defibrillator (AICD) implantation. Later that evening he complained of sharp pain in the left shoulder and left side of his chest. The post-implant chest X-ray is shown.

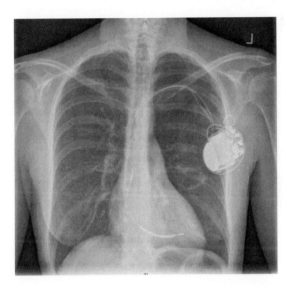

Questions:

1. What is the diagnosis?
2. What should be done immediately?

Answers:

1. Left sided pneumothorax.
2. Insert an under-water seal chest drain.

This obese 54-year-old man gave a six-month history of increasingly severe epigastric discomfort. Physical examination revealed no significant abnormalities apart from the hyperpigmented, hyperkeratotic, velvety plaques and papillomas on the back of his neck, shown below.

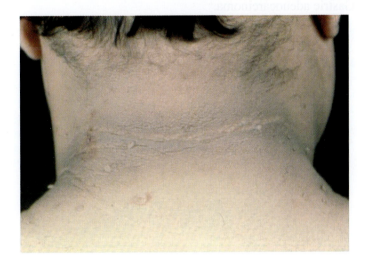

Questions:

1. What is the skin condition called?
2. Name the metabolic abnormality most associated with the condition.
3. What factor is responsible?
4. What investigation is most important here?
5. What serious associated pathology should be suspected?

Answers:

1. Acanthosis nigricans.
2. Hyperinsulinism/obesity.
3. Transforming growth factor-α — similar to epidermal growth factor.
4. Gastrointestinal investigations for malignancy e.g. gastroscopy. Diabetes — abnormal glucose tolerance test or raised glycosylated haemoglobin should be sought.
5. Gastric adenocarcinoma.

This 26-year-old lady presented with a three-month history of palpitations. Physical examination, ECG and echocardiogram were all normal. The chest X-ray is shown.

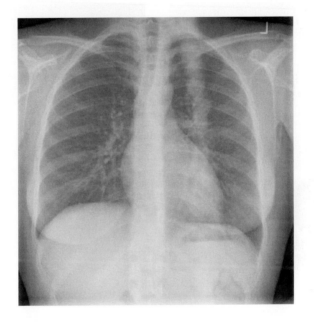

Questions:

1. What does the chest X-ray show?
2. What is the likely cause?

Answers:

1. An odd opacity running down the left hemithorax.
2. Her appearance shows the cause of the opacity to be an unusually long and thick plait of hair. With the plait held above her head, a repeat chest X-ray looks normal.

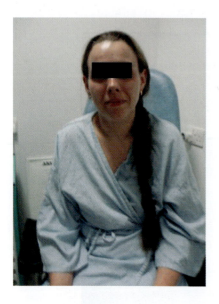
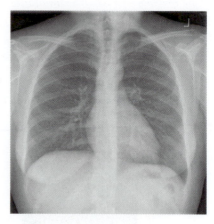

This young man presented with a six-week history of malaise and a two-week history of night sweats and intermittent rigors. He had become breathless on effort over the previous ten days and had developed painful tender spots on the palms of his hands and the soles of his feet. Physical examination revealed a pyrexia 37.8°C, pulse 100 bpm, an early diastolic murmur at the left sternal edge and palpable splenomegaly. The lesions on one hand and foot are shown.

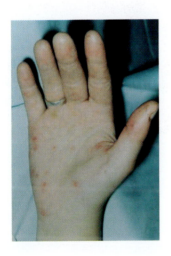
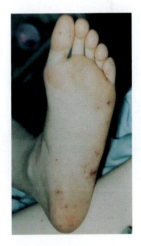

Questions:

1. What is the likely diagnosis?
2. What are the lesions on the hand and foot?
3. What four investigations should be performed initially?
4. What two other investigations are likely to be necessary?

David R Ramsdale

Answers:

1. Infective endocarditis.
2. Oslers nodes.
3.   (i) Blood cultures.
     (ii) Blood count.
    (iii) Chest X-ray.
    (iv) Transthoracic echocardiogram.
4.   (i) Transoesophageal echocardiogram.
     (ii) Cardiac catheterisation including aortogram.

Case 77

This 77-year-old man had undergone coronary artery bypass surgery 15 years earlier and permanent pacemaker implantation ten years after that. He presented with progressive pain and swelling in his left arm over the previous two weeks.

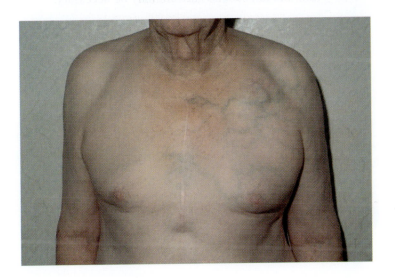

Questions:

1. What does the picture show?
2. What is the diagnosis?
3. What investigation would confirm the diagnosis?
4. What treatment is necessary?

189

Answers:

1. Dilated superficial veins over the left pectoral region, dilated external jugular vein and oedema of the left upper arm.
2. Left subclavian vein thrombosis.
3. Venogram of the left subclavian vein.
4. Anticoagulation with warfarin. If the symptoms fail to diminish over the next six weeks, explantation of the pacemaker and the leads within the left subclavian vein may be necessary.

This 18-year-old male presented with syncope and palpitations follow-ing a two day illness of diarrhoea and vomiting. There were no abnor-mal findings on physical examination. Haemoglobin 12.9 g/dL; white cell count 11 500/µL; serum sodium 133 mmol/l; potassium 3.3 mmol/l; urea 10.2 mmol/l; creatinine 110 mmol/l. The chest X-ray was nor-mal. The ECG during an episode of palpitation and syncope whilst being monitored on the coronary care unit is shown (top). A 12-lead ECG from his brother is shown below the patient's rhythm strip.

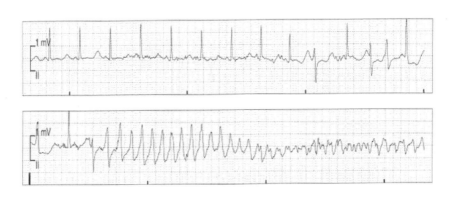

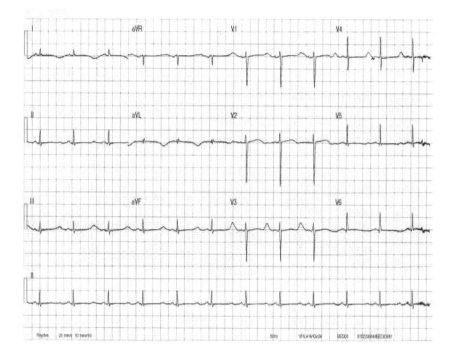

Questions:

1. What does the first ECG show?
2. What does the second ECG show?
3. What is the cause of the problem?
4. How should the patient be treated? What treatment would you advise for his brother?

Answers:

1. Sinus rhythm with a prolonged QT interval. Ventricular ectopic beats, R-on-T ventricular ectopic resulting in Torsades de pointes ventricular tachycardia.
2. Hereditary prolonged QT-syndrome.
3. Hypokalaemia due to the diarrhoea and vomiting.
4. Intravenous and oral potassium to correct the hypokalaemia, followed by elective implantation of an automatic cardioverter defibrillator (AICD). His brother should have an elective AICD implanted.

This 40-year-old lady developed pain over the lateral aspect of her right knee and lower leg. Within 24 hours a painful rash appeared (shown).

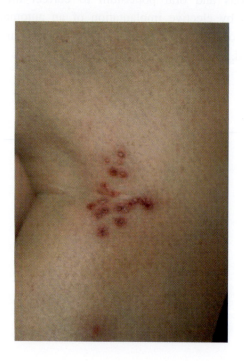

Q Questions:

1. What is the diagnosis?
2. What three treatments should be offered?

Answers:

1. Herpes zoster or shingles.
2. Paracetamol for pain relief. Acyclovir 800 mg 5 times daily for 7 days. Topical calamine lotion to dry the vesicles.

This 65-year-old man developed presyncope when carrying boxes during house removal. He had similar symptoms when hugging his wife (figures). An ambulatory ECG recording during an episode of severe dizziness is shown.

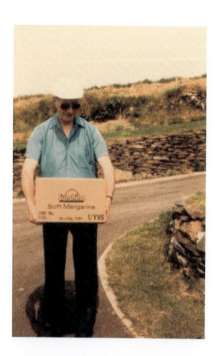
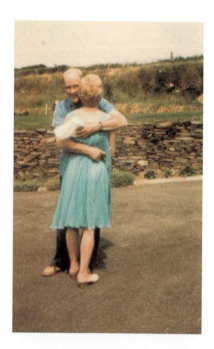

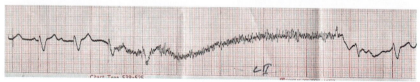

Questions:

1. What is the diagnosis?
2. What simple treatment is indicated?

A Answers:

1. Electromyopotential inhibition of a VVI permanent pacemaker in a pacemaker-dependent patient.
2. External reprogramming of his permanent pacemaker to bipolar sensing or VOO pacing is likely to fix the problem. This problem is infrequent now with the use of bipolar sensing pacemaker electrodes.

This 45-year-old lady complained of visual impairment. Fundoscopy is shown below.

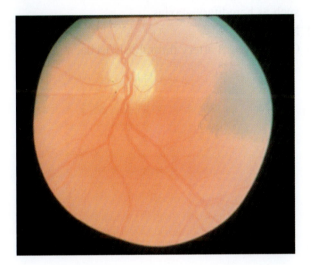

Questions:

1. What is the diagnosis?
2. Give five causes of the condition.

Answers:

1. Optic atrophy.
2. (i) Demyelination in the optic tract as in disseminated sclerosis and retrobulbar neuritis.
    (ii) Injury to the optic nerve or retina.
    (iii) Primary degeneration of optic nerve in heredofamilial disease such as hereditary ataxias.
    (iv) Methanol.
    (v) Central retinal artery thrombosis/ischaemia.

Case **82**

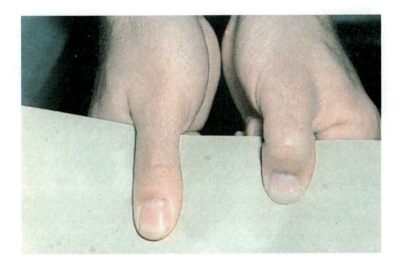

Questions:

1. What physical sign is being demonstrated here?
2. Which is the abnormal side and how is it physically abnormal?
3. What does this abnormality signify?
4. What muscles are affected by this lesion?
5. What can cause this lesion?

Answers:

1. Froment's sign.
2. The left hand thumb position is abnormal (right side of picture). It demonstrates the inability of the thumb to adduct and grip the piece of paper. The thumb therefore flexes in order to maintain its grip.
3. An ulnar nerve palsy.
4. A low lesion of the ulnar nerve causes wasting of the intrinsic muscles of the hand, with the exception of the outer two lumbricals and the thenar muscles other than adductor pollicis. Inability to adduct the thumb due to paralysis of adductor pollicis causes the thumb to flex due to contraction of flexor pollicis longus. A claw hand can also result with ring and little finger hyperextension at the metacarpophalangeal joints and flexion at the interphalangeal joints.
5. Injuries to the ulnar nerve can result from compression at the elbow, fractures of the medial epicondyle, penetrating injuries at any level, lacerations at the wrist or delayed palsy from marked cubitus valgus.

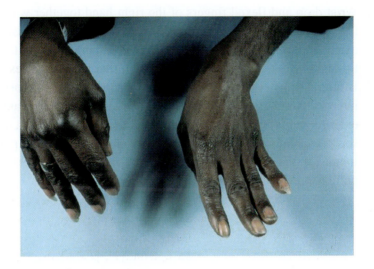

Questions:

1. What physical signs are evident?
2. What is the likely anatomical cause?

Answers:

1. Wrist drop and flexed fingers of the right hand together with failure to extend the left wrist on command. This patient was asked to extend both wrists. Only the last two phalanges are extended, through the action of the lumbrical and interosseous muscles.
2. Bilateral posterior interosseous neuropathy. The posterior interosseous nerve is a branch of the radial nerve and supplies extensor carpi radialis brevis, supinator, extensor digitorum, extensor digiti minimi and extensor carpi ulnaris, extensor pollicis longus, extensor indicis, abductor pollicis longus and extensor pollicis brevis.

This 26-year-old lady presented with sharp central chest pain made worse by inspiration, two weeks after an upper respiratory tract infection including a sore throat and myalgia. Her temperature was 38.1°C, pulse 118/min; JVP raised 5 cm above sternal angle. Haemoglobin 13.6 g/dL; white cell count 15 400/µL; ESR 98 mm/first hour. The ECG showed sinus tachycardia and the chest X-ray is shown. An echocardiogram was requested and is also shown.

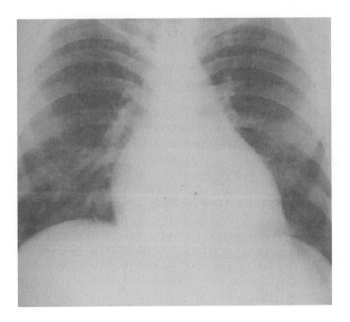

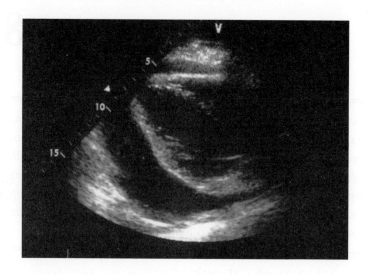

Q Questions:

1. What does the chest X-ray show?
2. What does the echocardiogram show?
3. What is the likely diagnosis?
4. What procedure is necessary?
5. What tests should be sought?
6. What treatment should be given?

Answers:

1. Marked "cardiomegaly".
2. Pericardial effusion.
3. Acute pericarditis.
4. Pericardiocentesis.
5. Pericardial fluid sent for microscopy, culture and sensitivity. Blood cultures. Serology for viral infection. Serology for autoantibodies.
6. Analgesia — paracetamol 1G 6-hourly; non-steroidal anti-inflammatory agent — indomethacin, ibuprofen or diclofenac. If effusion continues to recur, oral prednisolone 30 mg/day for first week; 20 mg/day for second week; 10 mg/day for third week and then reducing dose of 2 mg/week over next five weeks.

This 70-year-old lady complained of double vision.

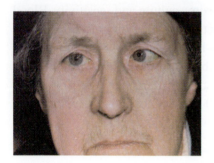 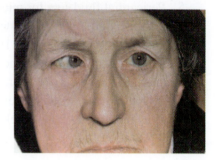

Questions:

1. What is the diagnosis?
2. What has she been requested to do during the physical examination?
3. What is the likely cause?

Answers:

1. Lateral rectus nerve palsy, following a road traffic accident — fracturing base of skull.
2. On the left, she has been asked to look to the right — right lateral rectus ineffective. On the right, she has been asked to look to the left — left lateral rectus ineffective.
3. Abducens or sixth cranial nerve palsy.

This 56-year-old lady complained of breathlessness after doing her housework and shopping, walking more than 200 yards or climbing stairs. Her symptoms had developed over the last three years and especially over the past six months. As a girl, she had suffered chorea and had a six-month period of bed rest in hospital. On examination, she looked well, pulse 100/minute irregular, JVP normal, BP 140/80 mmHg. Auscultation revealed a loud first heart sound, an apical mid-systolic murmur and a mid-diastolic murmur. She had mild ankle oedema. Her ECG showed atrial fibrillation. The chest X-ray is shown. An echocardiogram (recorded six months earlier) and cardiac catheterisation done during this admission are shown. The relevant haemodynamic trace is also presented.

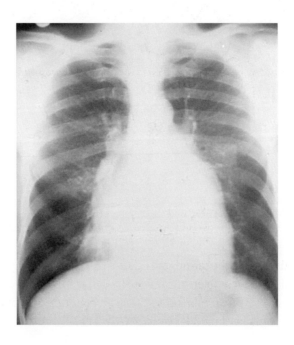

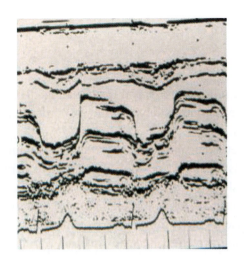

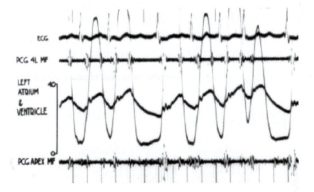

uestions:

1. What is the diagnosis?
2. What two features are present on the chest X-ray that are consistent with this diagnosis?
3. What does the echocardiogram show?
4. What does the catheter trace show?
5. What is the likely explanation for the recent deterioration?
6. What treatment should be considered?

Answers:

1. Rheumatic mitral stenosis and regurgitation.
2. Enlarged left atrium (straight left heart border); pulmonary venous congestion.
3. Poor leaflet excursion, flat top to the anterior mitral valve leaflet during diastole, fixed posterior mitral valve leaflet, dense echos from mitral valve leaflets due to calcification.
4. Mitral valve gradient in diastole of approximately 20 mmHg.
5. Recent onset of atrial fibrillation. Note that sinus rhythm is evident on the echo trace but patient was in atrial fibrillation at the time of cardiac catheterisation.
6. Mitral valve replacement. Surgical mitral valvotomy or balloon mitral valvuloplasty are inappropriate because of the evidence of a calcified, immobile mitral valve and mitral regurgitation.

Case 87

This 69-year-old lady complained of difficulty swallowing and painful blue fingers in cold weather. She smoked ten cigarettes per day and had a history of angina for 18 months. She was on atenolol 50 mg/day for hypertension and aspirin 75 mg/day.

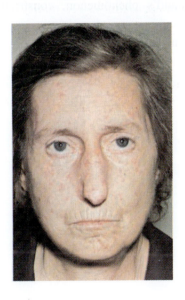 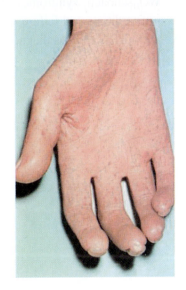

Questions:

1. What three features are shown by her face?
2. What does the hand show?
3. What is the diagnosis?
4. What other pathologies may develop?
5. What treatment should be offered?

Answers:

1. Fixed facial expression, small mouth, telangiectasia.
2. Fixed flexion deformity, sclerodactylia (acrosclerosis), digital ulcer/calcinosis at tip of middle finger, telangiectasia on skin of palm and fingers.
3. Systemic sclerosis or scleroderma.
4. Oesophageal stricture and dense pulmonary fibrosis (Thibierge-Weissenbach syndrome), Raynaud's phenomenon, constrictive pericarditis, renal failure, arthritis.
5. Steroids as soon as diagnosis is made.

Case **88**

This 50-year-old merchant seaman presented with this rash two weeks after returning from a voyage to Nigeria. This reddish papular eruption occurred mainly on the trunk and limbs and palms of his hands. On examination, he had a temperature of 37.6°C and he had cervical and inguinal lymphadenopathy. He had noticed odd itchy papules close to his anus.

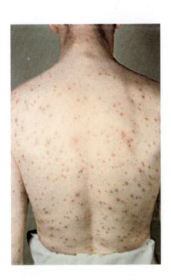 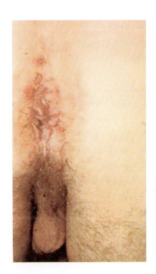

Questions:

1. What is the diagnosis?
2. What are the perianal lesions called?
3. What test should confirm the diagnosis?
4. What treatment should be given?

Answers:

1. Secondary syphilis.
2. Condyloma lata.
3. Non-specific initial tests: Venereal Disease Research Laboratory test (VDRL) or Rapid Plasma Reagin (RPR) test. Specific test: Fluorescent Treponemal Antibody Absorption test — FTA-ABS.
4. Benzylpenicillin G.

These itchy papules on the buttocks and genitals of this teenager were associated with similar excoriated lesions on the trunk and limbs, wrists and palms. The itchy rash was worse in bed at night.

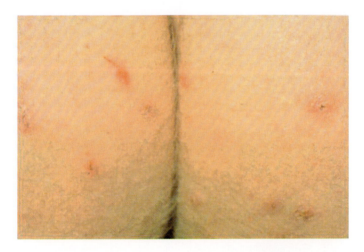

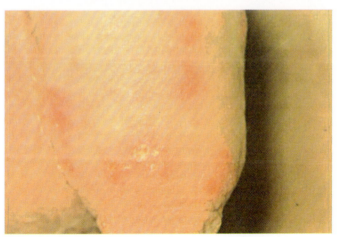

Questions:

1. What is the diagnosis?
2. What is responsible for the condition?
3. What treatment should be offered?

A Answers:

1. Scabies.
2. The insect/mite (acarus) *Sarcoptes scabei* variety *hominis* burrows into the keratin layer of the epidermis and lays her eggs. Active larvae then emerge and invade the adjacent epidermis. After 17 days, final male and female adult forms emerge. Copulation then occurs and the gravid female wanders over the skin and burrows once more to start the cycle again.
3. Hot bath followed by covering of body with emulsion of benzyl benzoate.

This lesion appeared on the chin of a young man whilst on a three-week holiday in the southern Mediterranean. Other lesions appeared on his forearms. They started as small papules, became scaly and ulcerated.

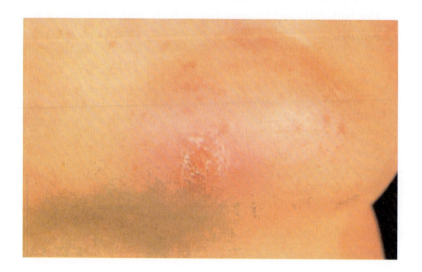

Questions:

1. What is the diagnosis?
2. What is responsible for the condition?
3. What is the vector?
4. What treatment is necessary?

Answers:

1. Cutaneous Leishmaniasis — causing the "Oriental Sore".
2. The protozoan, *Leishmania tropica*.
3. The Sandfly.
4. Often none as the lesions are self-healing. Resistant or recurrent lesions may require steroids/intralesional antimony.

This 65-year-old lady presented with breathlessness. She had had central chest pain three days earlier which had lasted 12 hours. She was reluctant to go to hospital. She had previously had a left nephrectomy, had hypertension and hypercholesterolaemia. On arrival, she looked pale and sweaty and was oliguric. JVP was raised 7 cm, BP 85/50 mmHg, heart rate 110/min and there was a pansystolic murmur at the left sternal edge. ECG showed sinus tachycardia, Q waves and ST-elevation in leads II, III, avF, V5 and V6. Chest X-ray showed pulmonary oedema. Cardiac catheterisation showed the following:

RA	17 mmHg	LV	77/18 mmHg
RV	49/20 mmHg	Ao	75/50 mmHg
PA	50/30 mmHg	PCW	22 mmHg (mean)

Oxygen saturations

SVC	32	IVC	29	RA	35	RV	85
MPA	84	rPA	85	LV	100		

Left ventricular angiography (LAO projection) is shown below.

Coronary arteriography showed an occluded RCA and mildly diseased LCA.

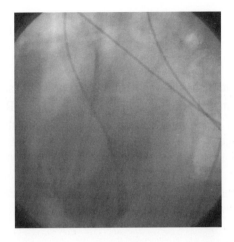

Questions:

1. What is the diagnosis?
2. What other test would have been useful diagnostically?
3. What medical treatment should be instituted?
4. What other treatment should be considered without delay?

Answers:

1. Inferior-lateral MI and post-infarct ventricular septal defect. The oxygen saturations suggest a large 4:1 L to R shunt. The LV angiogram (LV) shows contrast flooding into the right ventricle (RV) across the large VSD (arrow).

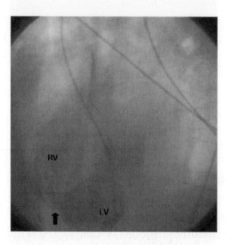

2. Echocardiography.
3. Insertion of intra-aortic balloon for counterpulsation — to help reduce the L to R shunt and improve coronary artery perfusion. Supportive inotropic agents. Possibly haemofiltration.
4. Surgical closure of VSD.

This young backpacker presented to hospital with a seven-day history of fever, headache, sweating and a maculopapular rash on his trunk that had spread onto his extremities. He had been hiking and camping through the forests of Indonesia. On examination, his temperature was 39°C, heart rate 118/min, respiratory rate 22/min and lymphadenopathy was evident. Chest X-ray showed interstitial pneumonia. The lesion below was noticed below his umbilicus.

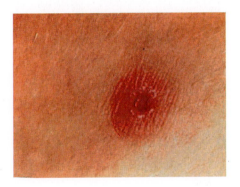

Questions:

1. What is the lesion?
2. What is the diagnosis?
3. What is the causal agent?
4. What is the vector?
5. What is the animal reservoir?
6. What test will confirm the diagnosis?
7. What treatment is indicated?

Answers:

1. Eschar lesion.
2. Scrub typhus.
3. The Rickettsia *Orientia tsutsugamushi*.
4. Mite (or chigger).
5. Rodents.
6. Positive blood culture for *Orientia tsutsugamushi*; increased titre of serum antibodies against *Orientia tsutsugamushi*; Positive INDX DIP-S-Ticks enzyme immunoassay dot test for detecting total IgG and IgM antibodies to *Orientia tsutsugamushi;* PCR on eschar sample material.
7. Azithromycin.

This 14-year-old boy walked into his mission school in Central Congo and was noticed to have these large sores on his left lower leg.

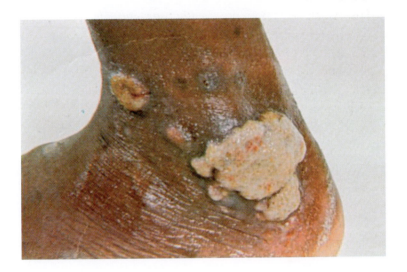

Questions:

1. What is the diagnosis?
2. What is the causal agent?
3. How is it acquired?
4. What treatment is indicated?

Answers:

1. Yaws.
2. The spirochaete, *Treponema pertenue*.
3. By direct human contact.
4. IM Procaine penicillin in oil. 1.2 MU given twice with an interval of 3–5 days.

This 23-year-old female presented with a four-day history of frontal headache and a 24 hour history of sudden weakness of her left arm and leg. There was no significant past medical history. Physical examination revealed a left hemiparesis with loss of power in the left arm and leg. There was an extensor plantar response in the left foot. The pupil in the right eye was smaller than in the left eye and there was a suggestion of ptosis of the right eye.

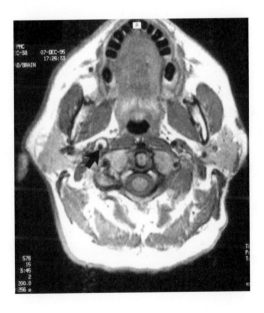

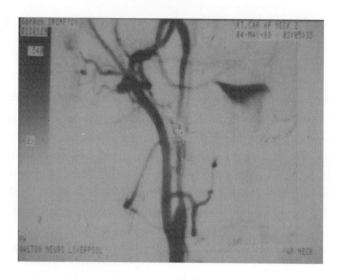

Questions:

1. What investigations are shown?
2. What is the clinical diagnosis?
3. What is the cause?
4. What is the aetiology?
5. What is the cause of the eye signs?
6. What treatment is appropriate?
7. What is the prognosis?

Answers:

1. MRI scan of head/neck; right carotid artery angiogram.
2. Ischaemia/infarction of right internal capsule.
3. Right internal carotid artery occlusion.
4. Dissection of the right internal carotid artery — shown as contrast/blood in false lumen of dissected ICA (arrow).
5. Partial Horner's syndrome — very suggestive of dissection due to local damage to sympathetic fibres which are wrapped around ICA in the neck.
6. Accepted treatment is 3–12 months anticoagulation to prevent embolic events.
7. Most dissections heal within 3–12 months and risk of recurrence is very low.

Case 95

A 35-year-old woman presents ten days after an uncomplicated delivery with a three-day history of increasingly severe headache, blurred vision, nausea, vomiting and drowsiness over the previous 24 hours. Physical examination revealed a drowsy, slightly confused lady with papilloedema. Before any investigations could be done, she had a grand mal fit from which she was slow to recover. Repeat examination then revealed a left hemiplegia. A CT scan and then an MRI scan of the head are ordered.

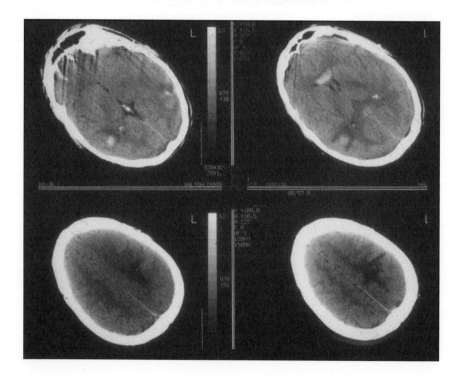

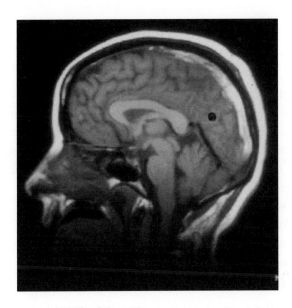

Questions:

1. What do the clinical symptoms and physical signs indicate?
2. Is lumbar puncture indicated here?
3. What does the CT scan show?
4. What does the MRI scan show?
5. What is the diagnosis?
6. What is the correct treatment?
7. Give three conditions that may be associated with this problem.

Answers:

1. Raised intracranial pressure.
2. No — lumbar puncture may lead to cerebral coning and death.
3. CT scan shows a "tight" brain with small areas of haemorrhagic infarction on the right and non-haemorrhagic infarction on the left.
4. MRI scan shows a thrombosed venous sinus which on MRV (Magnetic Resonance Venogram) fails to fill.
5. Cerebral venous/superior sagittal sinus thrombosis.
6. Anticoagulation with warfarin.
7. Post pregnancy, oral contraceptive pill, local or systemic infections, or tumour.

This 39-year-old man presented to the emergency department after an acute haematemesis. As the physician was about to insert an intravenous line in the antecubital fossa, she noticed the appearance below.

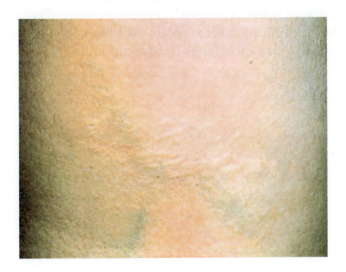

Questions:

1. What is the diagnosis?
2. What is the cause of the haematemesis?

Answers:

1. Pseudoxanthoma elasticum. The skin lesions are found most frequently at the sides of the neck, axillae, groin, cubital and popliteal
   fossae. Early in the disease, the cutaneous lesions are small, soft,
   chamois-coloured papules arranged parallel to skin lines and folds.
   Coalescence of these papules produces circumscribed or diffuse
   plaques which in advanced cases causes the skin to be thickened,
   loose and inelastic resembling the skin of a "plucked chicken".
2. This is an inherited disorder of connective tissue affecting mainly
   the skin, eyes and vascular system. Bleeding from the fragile blood
   vessels in the gastrointestinal tract occurs in 10% of cases and may
   be severe.

Case **97**

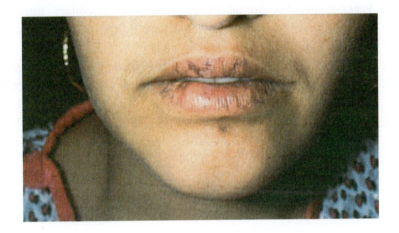

Questions:

1. What is the diagnosis?
2. How is it inherited?
3. What are the other main pathological findings in this syndrome?
4. What secondary features may occasionally be associated?

237

Answers:

1. Peutz-Jeghers syndrome. Also known as Hereditary Intestinal Polyposis Syndrome, it is evident here by the patches of hyper-pigmentation on the lips.
2. Autosomal dominant gene with variable incomplete penetrance.
3. Multiple hamartomatous gastrointestinal polyps which may bleed and cause anaemia.
4. Ovarian cysts, bronchial and nasal polyps, exostoses and clubbing.

This 30-year-old sheep farmer noticed an inflamed blister over the knuckle of his middle finger. It seemed to become blood stained before having the appearance below.

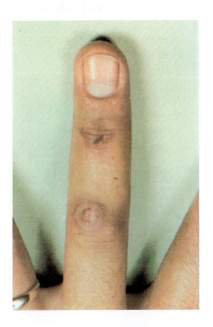

Questions:

1. What is the diagnosis?
2. What is the causal agent?
3. What are two other differential diagnoses?
4. What treatment should be given?

Answers:

1. Orf.
2. A pox virus.
3. Primary (accidental) vaccination, anthrax, erysipeloid.
4. No specific treatment. The lesion should resolve spontaneously.

Case **99**

A 33-year-old man arrived in the UK from Uganda with a two-week history of fever, widespread muscle aches and pain in his jaw. He had suffered an episode of diarrhoea just prior to becoming unwell. He thought that it was due to eating an inadequately washed salad/meat dish. On examination, he appeared unwell with a high, remittent temperature of 39.0°C, periorbital oedema and splinter haemorrhages under the nails of both hands. His muscles were tender to pressure and trismus was thought to be the cause of his jaw pain. Blood tests revealed eosinophilia.

The right deltoid muscle was particularly tender and a muscle biopsy revealed the likely diagnosis (shown).

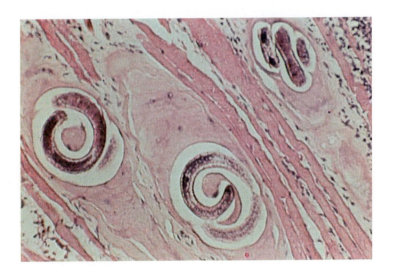

Questions:

1. What does the muscle biopsy show?
2. What is the likely diagnosis?
3. What is the source of the infection?
4. What other tests might confirm the diagnosis?
5. What treatment should be given?

Answers:

1. Cysts containing the coiled Trichina larvae are within the muscle.
2. Trichiniasis.
3. Infected pork.
4. Complement fixation test or precipitin test.
5. Thiabendazole is probably an effective antihelminthic for Trichiniasis.

This 78-year-old male with type II diabetes mellitus and hypertension over the last 6 years presented with sudden and almost total loss of vision in his right eye. It was preceded by "flashing lights and floaters" in the right visual field. Three days following the onset of symptoms, his vision was still markedly impaired in his right eye and limited to finger counting only. Opthalmoscopy revealed the appearance below.

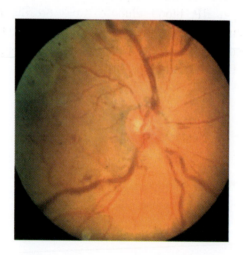

Questions:

1. What is the diagnosis?
2. Give three features shown on fundoscopy.
3. Name five risk factors that are associated with the condition.
4. What treatment is indicated?

Answers:

1. Central retinal vein thrombosis.
2. Hyperaemic optic disc. Papilloedema. Retinal oedema. Superficial haemorrhages, often scattered alongside the veins, which extend from the disc area out to the peripheral fundus. Tortuous dilated retinal veins with visible thrombus within them.
3. Age. Diabetes mellitus. Hypertension. Smoking. Hyperviscosity e.g. polycythaemia rubra vera, multiple myeloma. Raised intracranial pressure. Glaucoma.
4. Anticoagulants, thrombolytic therapy, aspirin and clopidogrel do not appear to be of much help. Check tests for associated systemic diseases e.g. BP, blood glucose, lipid profile, FTA-ABS, full blood count, viscosity studies, anti-nuclear antibodies. Serial opthalmoscopy is advisable as focal laser photocoagulation may be necessary for neovascular proliferation.